THE BEAUTY OF A SPIRAL

BETH MADDALENI

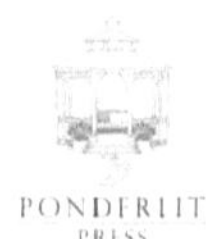

PONDERLIT
PRESS

AUTHOR WEBSITE: www.bethmad.com

Ponderlit Press
www.ponderlit.com

This story is a work of fiction and does not intend to offer advice or represent or identify any actual event, business establishment, facility, club, or person (alive or dead). Any real thing mentioned in this book is used fictitiously with products of the author's imagination. (See "Author's Note.")

COVER AND LOGO ART BY: Kaitlynn ("Katie") Jolley

Publisher's Cataloging-in-Publication data

Names: Maddaleni, Beth, author.
Title: The beauty of a spiral / Beth Maddaleni.
Description: Includes bibliographical references. | Saugus, MA: Ponderlit Press, 2023.
Identifiers: LCCN: 2023911315 | ISBN: 979-8-9881166-0-8 (paperback) | 979-8-9881166-2-2 (hardcover) | 979-8-9881166-1-5 (ebook)
Subjects: LCSH Figure skaters--Fiction. | Figure skating--Fiction. | Cancer--Patients--Fiction. | Friendship--Fiction. | Love stories. | BISAC YOUNG ADULT FICTION / Romance / General | YOUNG ADULT FICTION / Sports & Recreation / Winter Sports | YOUNG ADULT FICTION / Health & Daily Living / Diseases, Illnesses & Injuries
Classification: LCC PS3613 .A33 B43 2023 | DDC 813.6--dc23

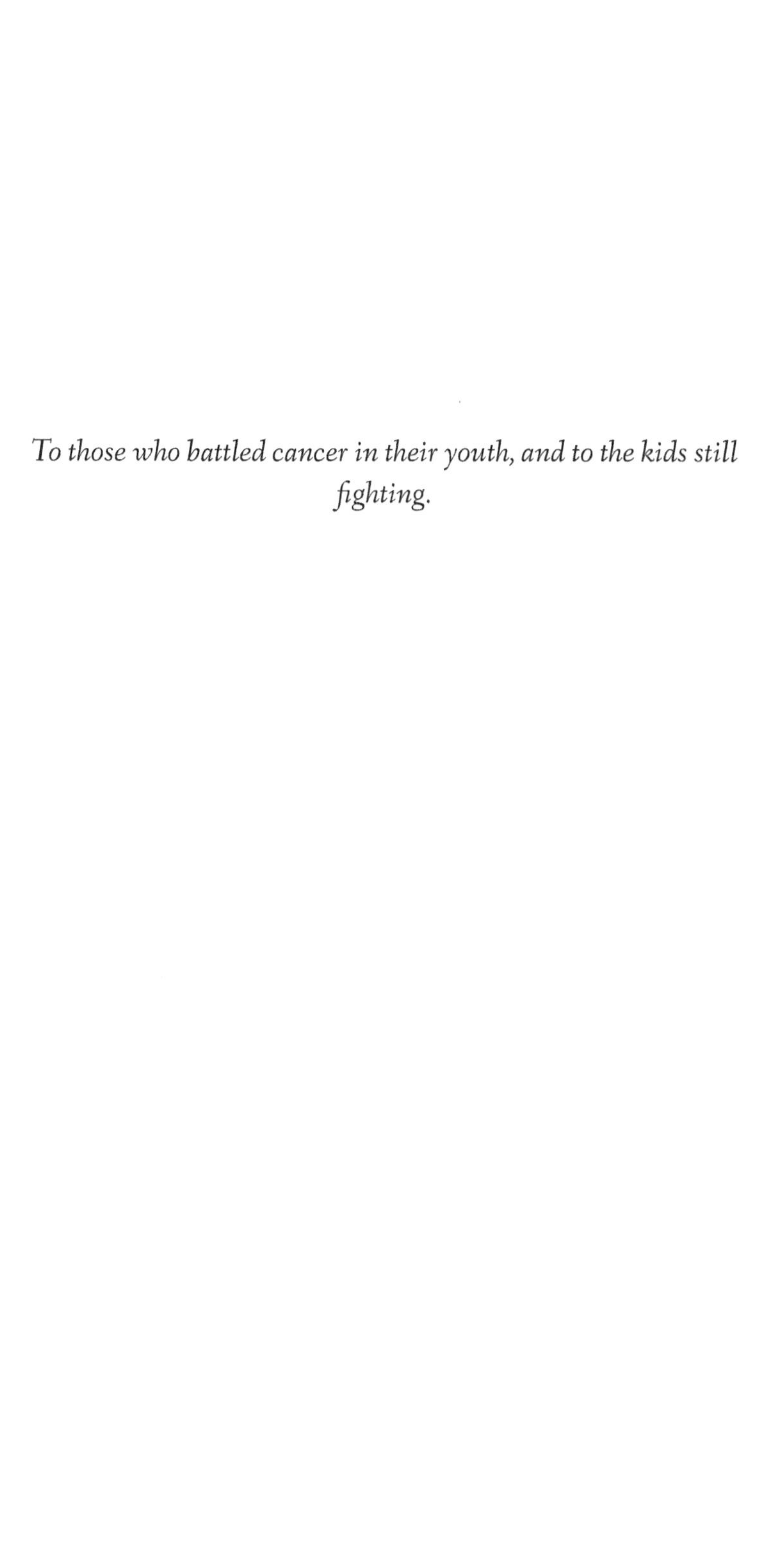

To those who battled cancer in their youth, and to the kids still fighting.

THE BEAUTY OF A SPIRAL

PART 1
"HARD FALL"

ONE

The day I left skating, I was sure of one thing: I didn't know exactly who I was other than a girl who hurt too much for her chronological age.

My blades sank into the ice, and each stroke, each edge, each three-turn resisted, forcing me to push harder. My program demanded more energy from me because the record-breaking end-of-May heat had leached into the rink, softening the ice. Instead of gliding across a smooth sheet, I slogged through a field of frozen fractals bent on gluing themselves to my blades. Out of energy, I still had to pull off a triple axel. *Double it,* I thought. On my worst day, I could land a double axel . . . until that day.

My right hip slammed into the ice. Panting, I rolled onto my knees, then stood up, hunching until I caught my breath. I looked up, and just as I had expected, my coach was shaking his head. Not a normal uh-uh shake. A slow you-pathetic-loser shake.

I mentally flipped him the bird and thought, *I'm not subjecting myself to this anymore.*

Instead of skating to my coach and completing my lesson, I hopped off the ice, hooked my guards on, and marched to the freezer humming by the lunch counter. There, I filled a plastic baggie with ice. Pressing it against my hip, I scurried into the locker room, tears stinging their way out of my eyes.

I reached into the side pocket of my skate bag and pulled out a tube of lipstick—red, the one I'd used for my salsa routine. I leaned against the counter, pressed my lipstick against the wall-length mirror, and wrote the following:

We spend all these hours here skating, beating up our bodies. I don't understand why. What's it all for?? A world exists outside these walls, where life involves more than ice packs + medals. Time to spread my wings + explore it. ~Madz

My mother would freak, but I'd made up my mind. I shouldn't have been this tired and sore at sixteen.

I removed my guards and tucked them into my skate bag. I wiped the water off my blades with a clean, dry rag, then repeated the process with a second clean, dry rag. Blades are beautiful things. Shiny, strong, and sharp (if they're taken care of properly), they hold an edge, a vital component of staying in control on the ice. Each jag on their picks is strategically sized to grip the ice for a perfect launch into a jump.

I held up my skate, slowly rotating it before my eyes as if it were a precious gem on display at Tiffany's. Every knick tells a story, but that day, all the stories merged into one: I'd beaten up them and myself for this sport. A tiny wedge of leather stuck up from the boot, so I pressed it back in. The damage had happened a week before, when my blade dug into the leather as I fell on an attempted quad toe loop. The slam contused the same hip I bruised five minutes ago.

At least I didn't fracture a vertebra like my best friend, Lindsey. It was a stress fracture caused by the repeated pressure her training had put it under. The problem came to a head seven weeks ago. Her body twisted when she fell hard after catching an edge on a rocker during her last maneuvers test.

I had a test to take myself, and I'd need to do it soon.

I slipped puffy terry-cloth covers over my blades, packed up the skates, and pulled out my phone. I searched the internet for local clubs hosting tests. The highest-level freestyle test would be my final figure-skating test. It would close this chapter of my life and launch the beginning of a new chapter.

I found a test session scheduled for the next day at a rink I was familiar with; however, applications were due two weeks before. Then I noticed the test chair was Lindsey's mother's best friend.

Call me as soon as you can, I texted Lindsey. *I need you to do me a favor.*

I peeked out the door to find Nathan coaching Joao. Nathan wouldn't waste the last few minutes chasing me when he could spend it coaching his star student, who'd won sectionals the year before and medaled at junior nationals.

"Hey," Lindsey said, peeking in, startling me. The rubber floor had cushioned her steps, silencing them. "When I left the gym, I saw you fall. Are you okay?"

"Yeah." I glanced in Nathan's direction. His focus remained on Joao.

She opened the door wider and held it open. "It looked like you walked out on your lesson with Nathan, but I know you wouldn't dare—"

"The session's almost over, and I'm skipping the next one. I'm tired, and the ice sucks."

"But I want to see your new program. You've skated on sucky ice before. Why aren't you looking at me?"

Cracking my knuckles, I looked up at her.

Her jaw dropped with a gasp. "You did walk out on your lesson." She peered at Nathan. "Aren't you afraid he'll block you?"

"I skated a session before lunch and a session after. Two out of three isn't bad, considering I wasn't going to come here at all."

She grimaced. "He's gonna block you."

Blocking skaters from texting or calling him was, still is, Nathan's *F-you*. For a few reasons, I didn't think he'd block me. For starters, he and my mother had a spiritual Type-A connection. They'd controlled my life in unison for the past six years, the harmony between them matching that of an Olympic pairs team: he'd dictate his life-controlling plan for me, and she'd religiously execute it, setting up my lessons, practice sessions, competitions, off-ice training, sessions with my choreographer, meetings with my nutritionist. Another reason, she'd always paid him and all involved in his plan on time. Finally, she's a powerful lawyer. Why burn that bridge?

"Let him block me. I have nothing to say to him anyway. Wait here." I grabbed my skating bag from the locker room, scurried back to the door, and cracked it open. "I have to get out of here."

"You're pale. I don't blame you if you'd rather relax by your pool. We're all vitamin D deficient around here. How's your appetite? Do you want me to grab you some juice? Maybe your blood sugar is low."

"I'm good, thanks." Eyeing the swinging doors leading to the main entrance, I deflected the conversation. "How's your back?" SuperEdge was like a nursing home. Around there, *How's your [fill in the blank]?* was the standard conversational courtesy.

"Better. The brace is off, and I'm taking Pilates classes to strengthen my core." She patted her abs. "I'll be back on the ice in a week. My mother says the new refrigeration system and doors will be in by then. With all the money this club takes from our parents, the ice should always be perfect."

I craned forward to make sure Nathan was still on the ice. "Did you get my text?"

"My mother has my phone."

My eyes lasered into hers. "I need a favor STAT. Call your mother's test-chair friend and ask her to squeeze me into her test session tomorrow morning. I'll text you a picture of my credit card."

She recoiled and shook her head. "No. Have you lost your freaking mind? You'll have to compete at the highest level, and no offense, you're not ready for that."

"I'm not worried about competing, but I would like to have something to show for all these years of training. Please. If you're my friend, you'll do it. Trust me. This is what's best for me. And no matter what, don't tell your mother until after I test. Otherwise, she'll tell my mother and sabotage my plan."

I stepped out of the locker room. "Beg the test chair if necessary. Or have her call me, and I'll beg her. Text me what she says." I hugged her goodbye. "When you have a day off, we'll have a pool party at my house."

As the Zamboni rolled onto the ice with its usual whine, the skaters hooked their guards on and scattered into the locker rooms. I scooted toward the door, hoping to make a clean break. My coach would have my butt on a platter for not skating the next session, not practicing everything we'd gone over during my lesson. At the moment, he was chatting with an off-ice trainer.

When the Zamboni plowed by Nathan, creating a temporary wall between us, I broke through the first set of doors, turned into the main office, and printed out a test application. I'd need signatures from a parent and a coach. Nathan would never sign it. I'd have an older girl I skated with a couple of years ago sign it. She coached at a nearby rink. I'd text her once I got in my car and have her sign it before I drove home, where I'd ask my father to sign on the parent's line. He wouldn't understand the significance of the test as my mother would. He attended my competitions and shows and often asked how my skating was going—that was it. Mom was the one who navigated my figure-skating career.

I broke through the final set of doors, into the sun, which instantly thawed my face and limbs. The rink wasn't frigid, but the contrast between inside and outside was stark. I threw my skate bag into the back of my SUV. As the liftgate closed, I turned, jumped back, and gasped.

"Where are you going? You have to run through your new program and work on . . ."

Gestapo. Jail warden. Possibly a warlock. These thoughts were not hyperbolic. When Nathan finished firing off the work-on list, I said, "My knee's bothering me. Don't wanna push it."

"Lie," he said.

"Truth," I snapped back. He was right, though. I was lying. Honesty wasn't the key to breaking out of this prison. Earlier, my honest complaint about the ache in my chest didn't stop him from pushing me. So I didn't expect him to give me time off for the freshly bruised hip and sheer exhaustion I suffered.

Lindsey's mother stared from the rink door. *Go in and worry about your own daughter*, my mind urged her, but the telepathic attempt failed. I was sure she'd already texted my mother. They reported to each other when one or the other wasn't at the rink.

"Those in motion tend to stay in motion and be successful," Nathan said, following me to the driver's-side door of my car. "Those who throw in the towel become inactive and tend to stay inactive. Inaction leads to a lack of success, not to mention soft, weak bodies. You'll become a soft, weak, unsuccessful person. And you're so much better than that."

"Thank you? But you know I've plateaued, and to be honest, I'm happy where I am. I'm just as happy landing a single axel as I am landing a double or triple."

"You rarely land a triple axel lately. It's only one more rotation, Madz, just one more. You've done it before, and you can do it again. Same with your triple toe loop. Even your quad. All you need to do to skate clean is focus, nail the required elements, and remember to breathe. And eat some protein. When I told you to lower your BMI, I didn't mean don't eat."

"I am eating." It had become impossible for me to keep up with the calorie count needed for his lessons and off-ice training. "And one more rotation on my end of this relationship could mean another stress fracture." Or worse, more blows to my mother's rink-mom ego. Which inevitably would mean more ice time for me, more off-ice training, more Pilates, more bruises.

"You haven't had a stress fracture since you were twelve, and the last I heard, your tibia healed and grew normally. Furthermore, you're missing the point. You've shined in the qualifying series before and placed at sectionals. If you could get back to where you were last year, you could win sectionals next year, and placing at nationals wouldn't be an unrealistic goal. But you need to persist. Falling on the double axel was just laziness. You gave up before you even took off."

"First of all, the ice was so soft it felt like my blades were carving through paste. Second, *you're* missing the point. You said not every skater peaks at 'best.'" I finger-quoted the last word. "I reached my peak; now I'm rolling backward. Besides, I've met my skating goals. I never said I wanted to medal at nationals."

"You told me you wanted to be the best."

"I was ten. I loved to skate. And let's face it: I'd been skating at a rink where it was easy to be the best. Most of the kids skated once or twice a week. SuperEdge turned what I loved to do into a job. Sometimes a bodily war. Tell me. Other than coaching or joining a show, where's all this skating going to take me, even if I were to win gold at nationals?"

"I'm doing very well coaching."

"But you've been stuck in a rink your whole life. Maybe I don't want that . . . no offense."

He twisted his lips and stared at me for a few seconds. "I have to go back in. I can't force you to practice, but if you don't, I'll have to let you go as a student. I have a waiting list of kids who want to work with me."

My point, I thought. Skating with him is work. A body-weakening job. Skating's supposed to be fun. Yes, it requires major effort, but it should instill a sense of joy and strengthen the physique, not wear it down. "Thank you for helping me become a really good skater, Nathan."

"What's that?" He took the test application from my hand.

I cracked my knuckles and bit my lip. He could find out in a minute when and where I was testing and run interception with the chair. If he found out Lindsey played a role in getting me into the test, he'd hold it against her. Bad for Lindsey because she wanted him as a coach. She was on his waiting list.

"I'm testing out. I'm done competing. Keeping my body intact is more important than medaling."

He paused, stared at me, then pulled a pen from his jacket and signed the paper. Handing it to me, he said, "Knock yourself out, Madz."

My jaw dropped. His hasty signing . . . hurt.

He turned his back on me and walked into the rink, ending our relationship. Nathan had one-upped my drama with a perfect execution of reverse psychology. Despite the impact, I wouldn't give in. I'd use his signature to my advantage.

For the first time since he became my coach, he wouldn't be at the test with me. *No biggie*, I told myself. I could hear him coaching me in my sleep.

Sleep. Something I looked forward to catching up on.

My stomach fluttered as I accelerated out of the parking lot. *I'm. In. Big. Trouble.* My mother might disown me. I'd severed my tether to this place, and I already felt myself whirling, my life spiraling out of control. Not because I regretted my decision. Because I didn't know what was next for me.

TWO

The day I left skating happens to be today. In my father's home office, I slouch in the cushiony leather seat in front of his desk, looking out the corners of my eyes at Mom. She stands in the doorway, frowning, arms crossed. You'd think someone died. Maybe someone did: the old me.

"Really, Madz?" she says. "You couldn't just tell Nathan you had cramps. You had to write a manifesto on the locker-room mirror."

I cringe when she mentions cramps around my father. "I wouldn't call it a manifesto."

Lindsey's mother is officially on my Ick List. The woman is a spy. Her test-chair friend is cool, though. She squeezed me into the test session and said I could pay at the hosting club's front desk tomorrow morning before testing.

"Don't you realize how lucky you are to skate at SuperEdge and have the best coach in Boston?" Mom huffs. "I'm utterly embarrassed."

"Mom. Please let it go. I'm sorry I let you down."

She enters the office and paces, a wineglass in one hand, a coaster in the other. "Someday you'll realize you let yourself down, Madz. Nothing happens unless you make it happen."

"I'll tell you what I made happen. I worked my butt off only to place third at sectionals last year and not even qualify for sectionals this year. I lost my triple toe. Today I lost my double axel. Do you know how hard it's been for me to subject myself to the SuperEdge walk of shame—from the rink to the locker room—every day for the past year? It's embarrassing." I try to shake the image out of my head.

"Practice makes perfect, and perfect is a Monroe tradition," Dad says.

Mom stops pacing and rolls her eyes.

Some may claim parents don't expect their children to be perfect. All I'd say to them is, "You haven't been to SuperEdge Rink and Skating Club." Where the adage *Kids should do a little better than their parents did* takes a back seat to *Kids should do at least as well as their parents*, most of whom are wealthy Ivy Leaguers.

"What's this B-plus in precalculus?" Dad asks, looking at the computer.

"I'm totally at peace with that B-plus." I'm so not okay with a B-plus. I was raised by two perfectionists. It rubs off.

Mom gulps a mouthful of Pinot Grigio. "He'll block us. I know he will. Listen to the message he sent me."

"No," I say.

"Ava," Dad says.

Mom places her wine on a coaster bearing the wisecrack *I only wine on days ending with Y*. She puts her readers on and holds her phone face-level. "Madz terminated her relationship with me today. It's been a pleasure working with her and you. Take care." She shakes her head. "So cold and permanent."

"I didn't say anything bad. I told him I was tired and would rather keep my body intact than kill it for a medal. Reasonable excuses."

She straightens her blouse and cracks her neck. "Okay. You're tired. We can work with that."

"Very understandable she's tired," Dad says, flipping through a construction contract. "Nothing a few good nights of sleep can't fix. She's still a growing girl."

Mom calls Dr. Weston. His office manager is used to squeezing me in under Mom's pressure. Health care is more urgent when your goal is the gold. Or, I should say, when your parents' goal is for you to get the gold. My parents' friendship with Dr. Weston and his wife also speeds things up. This appointment could screw up my plans.

Please not tomorrow morning, please not tomorrow morning, please not tomorrow morning . . .

Mom ends the call and tells me, "He'll see you late tomorrow afternoon. I'll leave work early to take you."

Whew.

"We can smooth things over with Nathan more easily if we present him with a doctor's note," she says.

The woman won't let go.

"Now get to bed," she says.

"I thought I might sit by the pool," I say.

"You said you didn't feel well," Dad says.

"I said I was tired. And I won't compete anymore. I refuse to waste another moment of my life killing my body and humiliating myself at the rink."

"You're exaggerating," Mom says. "You're not killing your

body. For God's sake, suck it up. All you need to do is attack your jumps with confidence. It's all about attitude."

"If it's so easy, why don't you do it?" Roughly eight out of ten SuperEdge skaters use this defense strategy. It has a 100 percent success rate. Parents can't seem to come up with a follow-up, and they won't pull us off the ice, sacrificing practice time and the money they invested into it.

"I hate when you say that." She lassoes her glass, rounds up another mouthful of wine, then plants the bulbous stemware on the coaster. "I don't even know who you are anymore. Where's my Madz?"

I grab a bottle of sparkling water from the little fridge under the dry bar. "When was the last time you fractured, twisted, or bruised any part of your body?" I turn to her with the cockiest expression I can muster up.

What's this? Her eyes are filled-to-the-rim pools. Quick breaths skip from her chest as she blinks out tears.

"I'm not lost, Mom. I'm right here." I point to myself. "See? No need to cry." My world has taken a turn into Locoville.

Ugh, now Gallagher, who's supposed to be dusting the bookshelves, gives me his famous look. He's our live-in butler, who's been here so long he's like family. Even saying "like family" doesn't sound right. He *is* family. You might wonder how an old guy with white hair, ruby cheeks, and bright blue eyes can appear anything other than cute. I'll tell you how. Add a twitch of an eye, a scrunching up of the chin, and exactly two rounds of head-shaking.

"I'll dust the shelves later," he says with his Irish brogue. He leaves the room.

Mom is a tough-as-Kevlar prosecutor capable of handling any level of sass—she has never cried over it. My skating is her

Achilles' heel. I know it; my father knows it. She takes her own walks of shame when I don't make it to the podium. By walking out on Nathan and SuperEdge, I've quadrupled that shame.

Truth be told, Mom's right. I've let myself down. If she were truthful with herself, I'm sure she'd admit there's something in my skating for her too.

Each of her tears pinches my heart. I wrap my arms around her and rest my head on her chest. "Thank you for everything you've done to support my skating. I'm just . . ." I sigh. Exhausted. Worn out. Beaten down. "Done." Had I stayed at the old rink Lindsey and I used to skate at, I'd probably be there now, energetic and skating with actual friends. My SuperEdge peers are more like coworkers. Deep down, they're probably relieved to cross me off their competition lists.

"When you're tired, it's hard to imagine doing everyday things." Mom kisses my head. "Dad and I get it." She breaks from my hug and dabs her eyes dry. "Now, I don't want to hear another word about giving up skating. I'm sure your outlook will change when you're rested and refreshed."

"She does look tired." Dad peers over his readers, analyzing my face. "She's pale too. I hope you have her eating more than just salads, Ava."

"She eats plenty of protein. Are you criticizing—"

"I have other news," I say, committed to dropping the mother of all truth-bombs. Although I'd rather not spark another argument, dropping this bomb will serve three purposes: (1) indirectly tell Mom rest won't change my outlook, (2) set the foundation for getting a test-application signature, and (3) ease the overall blow of my passing the test tomorrow. "I plan to take my final freestyle test. Soon."

Mom slaps her hand against her mouth. "But if you pass,

you'll have to compete at the highest level. You're not ready to compete at that level, at least not in qualifying competitions. You'll come in last."

Compete, compete, compete. "I've decided I'm not the competitive type."

"Ha!" explodes Gallagher from beyond the door. He usually doesn't provide commentary when my parents and I converse during his work hours.

He peeks in at me. I scrunch my face and peer at him, signaling him to stop fudging up my case.

"I'm going outside to take a nap," I say to my parents. In an hour, I'll sit with them for supper. That's enough time for them to absorb my confession and for me to refuel for the next round: squeezing a signature out of Dad for my test application. (The date line is blank.)

He stands and stretches while Mom follows me out of his office. As I head toward the French doors in the kitchen, destination backyard, I stretch my tight, achy neck and yawn.

"Wait," Mom says from the granite island. "I saw that. What's wrong with your neck?"

Dad hurries in. "What about her neck?"

"I fell hard. I bruised my hip, *again*, and probably pulled a neck muscle. We should ask Dr. Weston for a referral to the sports medicine clinic."

Mom throws her hands up and says to Dad, "No wonder she's discouraged."

"Makes sense," Dad says.

"Mom. Dad. I'm going outside to take advantage of the luxurious yard you've provided me with." All this stress, caused by unrealistic expectations and a lack of R&R. I open the French doors. According to the patio thermometer, the temperature outside has dropped to 74 degrees, so I shut off the AC and leave the doors open.

"Stop." Mom sweeps her perfectly angled blonde bob behind her ear. "You made a commitment to this sport. To Nathan. To yourself. To the club. Your father and I never expected you to get a job. Skating's been your job. Skating and school. Two things you need to finish.

"After you finish this skating season, you'll take your final skating test and compete at the highest level for at least a year. Your skating success will help you get into a good college and will light up your work resumé."

Says the woman who doesn't want to discuss this until I've gotten some rest.

"Have you forgotten? I'm a year ahead in school thanks to the online summer courses I've taken. I should be applying to college now, and I don't need to participate in more competitions to impress admissions officers or future employers. Once I pass my final skating test, I can tell them I completed a very intense program that required a long-term commitment and physical and mental stamina." All true, and a strong argument if I do say so myself.

"You told your father and me you were 'all in' with skating." She swigs her wine. "In response, we did everything we could to support you. You can't give up because you had one bad day. We expect you to finish what you started."

"One bad day? I've had a bad year. And for the record, I *am* finishing what I started. I wouldn't exactly call being gold-tested 'giving up.' It's a huge accomplishment." As long as I'm rested, my test will be a breeze. The hosting rink has hard ice, which sucks less energy out of me than SuperEdge's ice has lately. "If I don't take the test right away, I could get rusty and fail. Then I really would be screwed because I wouldn't go back to SuperEdge. Not to practice my test routine, not to tweak it if the rules change. No way."

My parents look at each other, telling me what's next. Mom says it out loud. "We don't support this decision. Taking your final freestyle test is not in your best interest."

I step onto the patio. I figured Dad would talk some sense into her, but he disappointed me. I glare at my mother. "You mean it's not in *your* best interest." Bragging rights. My purpose in life is to be a vehicle for her ego.

"Don't use that tone with your mother," Dad says.

My stomach knots, pushing up pure acid. "Okay. Sorry. And sorry we don't agree on my future in skating. Sorry for disappointing you."

I march across the patio, beyond the pool, and sink into the grass behind the poolhouse. A dandelion stares me in the face, defiant. I pulled one from the same spot last week. Soon I'm on all fours, picking more between nearby shrubs. "What do we have a landscaper for?"

With a handful of dandelions, I crawl back to the poolhouse and lie beside it on the cool, soft carpet of grass, too lazy to climb onto a lounge chair. My eyelids are as heavy as lead blocks . . .

CLIPPER-SNIPPING awakens me from my nap. I flick my eyes open, sit up, and scan the yard. I can't have a moment of privacy. With all the shrubs around here, he picks *that* rhododendron to trim.

"Nice to see you too," the landscaper says.

"Hi. Sorry. I've had a busy day." I wipe drool from the corner of my mouth, tasting a mixture of sleep and dandelion.

He points to the dandelions in my hand. "Those have medicinal qualities, you know. Some people actually make an effort to grow them."

Sleepy breath, sleepy face, sleepy hair, no makeup. I'm not conversing. Not even to tell him that as our landscaper for the past year, he's to blame for the weeds springing up in my yard. Standing, keeping my head down, I say, "Nice to see you—have a good day," and scurry away.

Don't say anything, don't say anything, don't say . . . Why didn't he say anything? I finally have time to go on a date with him, and he stops asking me out. Whatever.

"I heard your parents talking. The door's open."

Ugh. I stop in my tracks and turn to him.

"Your mother said she won't pay for your test, whatever that means." He returns to clipping. "Should I start a Please-FundMe account for you?"

"What are you talking about?"

"You know more about it than I do. I'm just telling you what I heard. She said she's going to cancel your card."

"My card?" I gasp. My credit card. Knowing I plan to test soon, of course she'd execute a hostile maneuver to regain the upper hand. This debacle could stop me from testing tomorrow.

I toss the dandelions into the trash and head to the kitchen. My parents have more money than they know what to do with. I knew Mom was a control freak, but no. Not this. She wouldn't.

THREE

Both of my parents sit at the kitchen table, quiet. Not a good sign. I'll check my credit-card status after dinner. I offer to help Gallagher, but he says he's all set and serves the food. He acts as if it's an average day because, well, he's like that. He's been living with us since I can remember. Other than the occasional *Ha!*, he doesn't usually "break character" until after dinner.

Mom says Gallagher's the epitome of professional. "He goes above and beyond," she's always said. He cooks, cleans, and before I got my license, he'd drive me to the rink while my parents worked. I like him because he's sweet in an Irish grandfather kind of way. He doesn't talk much, but he's got a calmness about him our house eats up. Which is why I put up with his occasional eye-twitching, chin-scrunching, head-shaking "look."

I'm starving for an appetite, but I eat anyway. Good nutrition is a must if I'm to pass my test, no matter how easy it should be to pass. I plan to take it regardless of my credit-card situation. My parents haven't mentioned a word about it, but the air is tense. Judging from the muscle-twitching in Mom's jaw, she's holding back an inevitable conversation.

When I finish dinner, Dad leans forward in his seat. "Madelyn. Your mother and I . . ." He eyes her and shakes his head. She nods, prodding him to continue. "We can't pay—"

"Won't," Mom says. "We won't pay."

He sighs. "We won't pay for your final test. I'm sorry. It's not in your best interest, dear. It just isn't."

Neither is financial sabotage. "My test is tomorrow, first thing in the morning." This is crunch time. Truth time. Emboldened by the presence of Nathan's signature, I slap the application on the table. "It's at—"

"We figured out when and where you're testing," Mom says.

I doubt Lindsey's the snitch. I've kept too many of her secrets for her to rat me out. "You talked to Lindsey's mother," I say, "which is why you came home early. She called you after hearing about me from her test-chair friend." How naive of me to have assumed the test chair wouldn't gossip.

"It doesn't matter how I found out. The bottom line is you're not taking the test. I canceled your credit card as a precaution. We gave it to you strictly for food, gas, and an emergency. Since you'll be home until you find a job, you won't need it. And now that I have the test chair's phone number"—she holds up a slip of paper—"I'll make sure you don't test tomorrow."

Dad shifts in his chair.

Passing my final freestyle test would be a huge accomplishment despite its negative effect on my competitive career. Why would my own mother stop me from taking this test when I'm most prepared for it? I press my napkin against my mouth as if such a thin barrier can stop me from going full throttle on her.

I uncover my mouth and release the words backing up in my throat. "I will never. Ever. Ever. Skate again. *If* you tell the test chair I can't test. Nev. Er."

I run outside, leaving my test form on the table. I doubt Mom will rip it up with Nathan's signature on it. If anything, she might take his cue and sign it, gambling on reverse psychology. My phone buzzes with a text from Lindsey: *I'm sorry my mother ratted you out. The freaking test chair told her what happened.*

Me: *It's not your fault. Still gonna take the test. TTYL*

One tiny problem: where do I get the money?

I'm not much of a saver. Never had to be. When I ran out of the money I earned from teaching group classes, my parents gave me money or bought me what I wanted. Spring group classes are over, and summer group classes haven't started yet. I'm broke. No longer the perfect child, I'll stay broke unless I get a job.

I have no time to sell anything, not that I have anything I want to sell. I donated things I'd lost interest in or outgrew. Everything I currently own, I want: car, electronics, skates.

My nosey landscaper is clipping the hedges by the side-yard entrance, so I dart across the backyard and hide behind the poolhouse again. Panting, I lean against it, slide to the ground, and close my eyes. Clutching the grass, grounding myself, I take a deep breath that fights through an ache in my chest. I purse my lips and exhale slowly, determined to calm myself. A meltdown will fray my nerves and confidence, causing me to slip up on my test.

Ugh. Please no. The clippers close in on me with a vengeance. I can't even thwart a meltdown without having my personal space invaded. Worse, he's cute. Worse than that? This kid always sees me at my worst. Always. After skating, after off-ice training, after Pilates. Never a break. He must think I don't own a brush or deodorant.

"I know it's none of my business," he says.

I tilt my head up, squint, and speak to his back. "Apparently, my parents have this thing about using money as a weapon. They want me to change my mind about something."

He stops clipping, turns to me, and raises his brow. "And that something is?"

"They don't want me to take my final skating test. They're convinced rest and a doctor appointment will change my mind." His worn work boots add a touch of rugged attractiveness to him.

"And they're using money as a weapon by . . ." The sun-bronzed clippermeister resumes his clipping, shaping an arborvitae.

"Not paying for my test." Why did I blow my birthday money on a scooter I had no time to use? (I gave it to Lindsey's brother.)

The landscaper stops clipping and turns to me again. "Why is taking your skating test a bad thing?" A loop of his dark-brown mane dangles over sweat beads on his forehead.

"Taking this particular test means I'd have to compete at the highest level."

He resumes clipping. "And competing at the highest level is bad because . . ."

"I'd take a total butt-kicking. Competitors perform way more difficult moves than their test level requires." Lately, I've barely been able to meet the competitive requirements for my current level. "In a nutshell, the test signifies the end of my competitive-skating career. My parents aren't ready for that yet."

He pauses his clipping. "Hmm . . ."

Breathe in; breathe out. Try not to look ugly. The wind blows strands of hair not locked into my ponytail, and I blow the wisps out of my face. They fall right back down on it.

He resumes clipping. "Does this mean you're joining the rest of us in the real world?"

I pick the wind-blown strings of hair from my mouth—"I guess it does"—and tuck them behind my ear. "But I'm kinda screwed if I can't take the test ASAP." I hug my knees. "If I wait, I'll get rusty, and the test rules could change, forcing me to adjust my program." Talk about the prolonging of agony. I'd need to find a coach and spend more time on the ice—if I could stand it—nulling and voiding my dramatic exit from the rink today. "I've worked too hard in skating to miss this chance to take my final test now, when I'm ready."

He lowers the clippers, turns to me, and twists his adorable lips.

"Why are you looking at me like that?" I re-tuck the wild wisps behind my ears and break eye contact.

"I have a proposition for you," he says.

Yes. I will go on a date with you. I'd relish an opportunity to show him I know how to groom myself.

"Did you hear me?"

I look up at him. "Yup. Propose away." Two months ago, I refused his Sunday-afternoon movie offer because I had to teach two private lessons. (I spent the money I made on a new workout outfit.) The last time he asked, last month, I was heading out of town to see a competition.

"I'll pay for your test. I figure that will fix"—he waves a hand toward me—"whatever *this* is."

"What you're witnessing is meltdown prevention." God, he's cute. With the tiny arborvitae branch sticking out of his hair, he looks like a tree warrior. "Do you realize the cost? We're talking a hundred and fifteen dollars. Can you afford that?"

"A hundred and fifteen? I thought those tests were thirty-five plus a small hospitality fee."

Admiring the rhododendron he trimmed earlier, I say, "The lower test levels are cheaper. Plus, on top of the hospitality fee, I have to pay non-member and late fees. In the perfect world, I'd have an extra twenty-five dollars for practice ice, to warm up for the test." With a sudden realization, I catch his eyes again. "Wait. How does a landscaper know the going rate for a skating test?"

"We're making a deal, not holding an inquiry." He rests the clippers on the grass, takes a wad of cash from his pocket, and pulls out a Benjamin, two Jacksons, and a Hamilton—one hundred fifty dollars. "The perfect-world scenario plus ten extra for unforeseen expenses. But you have to pay me back in the form of lessons. Lessons for my sister, not me."

"You have a sister who skates?" I don't know his name, much less he has a sister.

"Yes," he says. "She wants to compete. We had to drop her coach because she went up on her rates, and ice time is expensive. It was too much for my budget."

"*Your* budget? How come—"

"It's not an inquiry, remember?"

Why his parents' budget is missing from the equation will have to remain a mystery. What shouldn't be a mystery? His name. My not knowing it is a direct result of all the running around I've done. Or running into my house when he came to landscape, avoiding him because I looked like I do now.

When he asked me out, I thought he was joking. Both times I was a raggedy mess from training. Maybe he doesn't ask me out now because the disaster before him isn't a joke anymore; it's just plain sad.

"I'll give her two lessons, each an hour long." Too much time has gone by for me to ask his name. Must be obvious I don't know it. I'm too embarrassed to ask.

"Four one-hour lessons or no deal." He holds up the money. "I'm being very generous, considering the emergent nature of the loan, which technically should warrant bonus lessons."

"Three hours. Still well under my worth, and it's all I can handle right now. I need to catch up on six years' worth of sleep." And *hel-lo*, I'm done with skating rinks.

"Okay, but in lieu of a fourth hour, she gets to borrow a competition dress of her choice from your closet. She's about your size. Not quite as slim, but those things stretch, don't they?"

Easy one. "Yes, they do stretch, and I'll go a step further. I'll give her lifetime access to my competition-dress closet. I have practice dresses and test dresses, too, if she needs them." I was ten pounds heavier when I wore most of them. "But remember. This deal's about my giving her my best in a specific amount of time. I'm not a miracle worker, so I can't guarantee results. If she doesn't progress, that's on her."

"Deal." He holds out his dirt-stained hand, and I shake it.

"What level does she skate at?"

"She passed her pre-tests, but she's kinda—never mind. We'll cross that bridge when we get there. Now, rest up. You have a test to pass." He hands me the money.

His stomach growls as he picks up his clippers and goes back to work. I run to the house and ask Gallagher to bring the landscaper a glass of iced tea and a plate of food. I plan to run through my test program and practice my jumps off-ice. Thanks to my new business partner, I have an important test to take tomorrow.

FOUR

"Marilyn Monroe, please take the ice," a microphoned voice echoes through the rink.

WTF. I hop onto the ice and stroke to the center, my starting point. Brown hair, brown eyes, small boobs. Do I look like Marilyn Monroe, lady? Deep breath, pose. I break character and glance at the judges. They're stone-faced. I'm usually more focused, but someone just fudged up. They should know my real name; I've tested here enough times.

"Excuse me. Madelyn Monroe."

The music starts, and I push off. Back straight, shoulders square, I bend my skating knee and stretch my free leg with each stroke, gliding across the ice as if my blades are set on autopilot, driving me through the required elements. I'm on a mission, and nothing's going to stop me.

Breathe. My chest aches a bit on the inhale, but I'm . . . *exhale . . .* okay.

I turn onto a back outside edge and jump into, land, a

double loop. I push against the ice as fast and hard as I can, footworking into a spread eagle, my entrance for a double Lutz.

Next on the agenda is a flying camel. I spin centered and fast, two more revolutions than required. I exit the spin, throw in a few flowing maneuvers, and gain momentum. Then I point my right toe, push into a three-turn, vault off the pick straight up into a double flip, land, vault into a double toe loop, and check out. That's how a double-double's done, my friends.

My edges propel me across the length of the rink, clinging to every curve, swerve, rocker, choctaw, and twizzle. Before you can say, "Phenomenal step sequence, Madz," I pull off a single axel and center a Biellmann spin.

I was once able to get through a routine like this and barely sweat. Now, I'm huffing and puffing, my steam fizzling out. I inhale deeply, blow it out, inhale again. *Please give me this, God.* Physically, I'm a lightweight, but fatigue is weighing me down. Adding more weight, Mom's absence. The realization saddens me. She has always come with me when I tested.

Making matters worse, I'm skating to "Ave Maria," a musical rendition of the Hail Mary. It's the violin version, but I know the words and their meaning by heart, and today they hit too close to home. Fortunately, I'm setting up for a spiral. The simple move will give me a break for a few seconds. I inhale deeply. On the exhale, a tear escapes me.

I simultaneously push onto my left foot, raise and extend my right leg, arch my back, and pull back my arms. As I glide on my outside edge, the tear clings to my cheek, quivering in the wind. I sail past the judges, catching the eye of one. She cracks a subtle yet distinct smile.

The beauty of a spiral isn't just its form or that it gives you time to breathe. It gives you a chance to take in your surroundings. To snare, in a milli-speck of time, a smile or an encouraging nod that sparks the confidence you need to get through this kind of test. Especially important when you're testing alone, without the blessings of your parents.

I mohawk into a split jump, land, step into a right inside three-turn, and launch into a double toe. After picking up speed with crossovers and footwork, I step down on a back outside edge and lift off for a double loop–double loop combination jump. *Yes.* Landing it is a huge deal because I'm nearing the end of my program. My gas gauge is creeping in on empty.

I suck in another deep, achy breath. *God, please give me the next jump too.* I gain momentum again with more stroking and crossovers, then position onto a back left inside edge, bend, and thrust myself up—into a double Salchow—and check out. The Lord had mercy and grew me an invisible pair of wings.

The ice and my blades cooperate as I step onto a forward left outside edge and curl into a sit spin . . . step down on my right foot into a back sit spin . . . and rise from it, holding and extending my leg over my head for the rest of the combination spin.

I end my routine with a centered layback, spinning without traveling—I can feel it. I straighten my torso, holding on to the spin and my center until the music's about to end. I pick the ice with my free foot, swirl to a bow, then straighten out, gracefully pulling my arms back and lifting my chin. I hold my pose for a beat, then slowly raise my right arm, guiding the last precious musical note to Heaven.

I break character and skate to the judges.

"You're all set," one says.

"Thank you," I say, forcing a smile.

The room dims to gray, and I'm pretty sure the lights are

only going out in my head. I reach for the sideboard and let it guide me off the ice. Hungry for air, my lungs devour a deep breath. I sit on the bleachers, catching my breath. Bending over to unlace my skates brings the blood back to my head.

A fresh tear splashes onto my hand, and my nose stuffs up, but it's okay. I'm having an epiphany: I don't totally suck at skating, and I'm still capable of harvesting joy from it.

That revelation lessens my guilt over Mom signing the test application. After making the deal with the landscaper, I grabbed the form from the table, ready to stomp into my father's office and beg him for his signature. I stopped in my tracks at the sight of her big, swirly John Hancock. I guess I have Nathan to thank for that. Without his signature on it, hers wouldn't be there.

I've been able to perform the elements of my test for years. It's the triples and quads that have been killing me lately. Except for yesterday, when a double axel did me in. Of course, my clean skate today doesn't create the possibility of placing at a significant qualifying competition. But I do think if I weren't so worn out, I could place in a local qualifying one.

I worry if I made the right decision. Did I do the right thing, testing out?

A runner hands me my test result. I passed. Comments include: elegant facility, strong edges, spins well centered and fast, good height on jumps, gorgeous spiral. The last comment flatters me most because the spiral, when performed correctly, is an element that many people enjoy watching for its elegance.

Packed up and ready to go, I beeline it to the bathroom, close the stall, and bawl. All those hours training. All the aches. All the visits to sports medicine and physical therapy. All the pressure of testing up and competing at a higher level. All the good moments, too: spinning, landing triples, and once, landing a quad toe loop. Hanging in the air, defying gravity—I love that sense of flight.

I forgot skating could make me feel so confident, so sure I was born to do it. But the thought of spending hours upon hours skating and training . . . I barely had the energy to get through this test. And I long to experience things I've daydreamed about: normal things, like spending summer days at the beach or in my backyard with friends, swimming, eating ice cream. If only I could rest this weary body of mine and heal its aching parts.

"Madelyn? Are you okay?" Test-chair lady's voice echoes beyond the stall.

"Yes, thank you. Tears of joy." A weird chuckle-hiccough erupts from my throat, the grand finale of this awkward conversation.

When she leaves, I peek out the bathroom door. The coast is clear, allowing me to bolt out of the rink and avoid being more of a spectacle than I've already been. These people know the deal. They know I'm an elite SuperEdge skater who has veered off course by "testing out" of the competitive circuit.

I burst through the doors, and the sun splashes my face, melting the cold off my skin.

"Hey." My imagination has me hearing the landscaper's voice. Can't be. I'm fifty minutes away from home. "Madz." This is not happening. My makeup has turned into facial spin art from all the crying. Can't this kid time an appearance when I'm *not* a mess? I speed-walk, but he catches up to me.

"I didn't think being stalked was part of our deal." Head down, I press my fingers under my lower lids and wipe, hoping to erase the mascara stains.

"This isn't stalking. I'm seeing how my investment worked out."

I thought I liked this kid. "You didn't invest. I'm paying you back, remember?"

"How'd you do?"

"I passed." I throw my skate bag into the back seat—no time to play around with the liftgate. I hop into the car, lock it, and steal a glimpse in the mirror to see if he's in the rearview. He's not. He's knocking on my window. I roll it down. Congratulations, cute landscaper, on having an up-close-and-personal view of Madz's makeup apocalypse.

"Congratulations." He passes me a single rose, and a smile blooms on my face. I've always gotten flowers or some other present—a new cell phone, for instance—when I passed a test or competed. That said, it's not just the rose making me smile. I wasn't as alone as I thought I was. He showed up.

I sniff the rose and look up at him. "Thank you."

Our eyes interlock. "You're welcome. And thank you in advance for giving my sister a lesson today. She's looking forward to it."

Did he say *today*?

A deal's a deal, and if I go today, I'll get one out of three lessons out of the way. "Which rink and what time? Can't be too late. I have an appointment at four thirty. Oh, and usually, coaches have to pay a fee."

"Already took care of the fee, and she skates at one o'clock. She has a half-day of school today." Smiling, he hands me a slip of paper with his sister's name and the rink's name. Several minutes north of Boston, it's a few miles away from my house. I skated there before going to SuperEdge. Cute Landscaper departs. Rolling up my window, I track him until he drives off in his pickup truck.

I blast the AC. After a morning test, Mom usually takes me to the pancake house, where I get the combo: scrambled eggs and a slice of French toast topped with raspberries. Now, just the thought of eating nauseates me. I uncover the yogurt I packed and swallow a spoonful. A sharp pain shoots through the right side of my neck, and I reflexively touch the spot that panged. My fingers land on a lump over my collarbone. I thought it was a pulled muscle when I first felt it last month. Distracted by my busy schedule and other aches, I forgot about it until now. It has grown from barely noticeable to almost the size of a golf ball. Weird.

FIVE

By stepping through the doors of this crappy rink, I've taken a few steps backward, into skating purgatory. "Why is this place so dingy?" I say under my breath. Super-Edge may have a glitch in its refrigeration system, but it's otherwise modern, not a dinosaur like this dank rink.

I passed my final test, I tell myself. The thought washes away my annoyance over being here. Another thought plants a smile on my face: *I'll be skating on my own terms after fulfilling my commitment to Cute Landscaper.*

I sweep on a fresh coat of lip gloss and keep my chin up as I enter the rink area. While passing a locker room oozing a pungent bouquet of dirty socks and sweat, I hold my breath and wave back to familiar coaches waving to me. I took group lessons from them in kindergarten and first grade. My former private coach isn't here, but Lindsey's is. We wave to each other. How can she stand showing up at this place all week?

These kids are a mess. Their skating, that is. Their arms are all over the place, and their picks take out chunks of ice when they jump. I substitute-taught several times for Nathan and other SuperEdge coaches, giving private lessons to skaters under my test level. None of them skated this poorly.

A girl about my size, slightly heavier (a healthy slim), skates over, waving enthusiastically. She's wearing a pink dress that fits Cute Landscaper's description. She resembles him—dark hair, similar eyes—but her cheeks are rosier than his, her skin fairer. Her hair's in a lopsided ponytail, wisps flying around worse than mine did when I bartered with her brother yesterday.

She bangs on the plexiglass panel.

Oh, no. I goggle at the sight despite wanting to turn and run away. *Please stop,* I try to telepathically convey to her.

I swivel my head toward Lindsey's former coach. Her eyes flit from me to the girl, to me again, and she rolls them. Message received. I'm about to teach a rabble-rouser. I wonder if this coach heard about my sudden exit from SuperEdge. *Ugh.* I wonder if she heard about my lipstick "manifesto."

I signed it confidently, sure my message was a necessary PSA that could prevent others from throwing away their lives and health. Now I wish I'd left it unsigned. If these coaches or the proctor heard about it, they could view me as a rebel and refuse to let me coach on their ice. Teaching a scene-maker won't help my case.

The girl in pink skates by the boards, shadowing my walk to the bleachers. I smile and nod, trying to project calm. She doesn't get the hint. She bangs the plexiglass again, points to herself, and nods, signaling, *Hey, look at me. I'm the one you're teaching.*

I'm a low-key kind of girl. Technically, even my abrupt

retreat from SuperEdge was low-key. A pantomime would have made more noise than I did. So yeah, this chick had better turn the volume down.

I spot Cute Landscaper walking from the proctor's booth to the bleachers. He grins and waves to me.

His sister pokes her head out of the rink. "You're late. The session started five minutes ago."

Great. I gave up Nathan to get a student who watches the clock as closely as he does. "Are you Gracie?"

"Yes. And you're Madelyn Monroe. I found pictures and videos of you on the internet."

"That's me. Nice to meet you." I finish lacing my skates and step onto the ice with the Pink Detective. Her pink scrunchie, pink dress, and pink gloves match her pink cheeks. "Can you stroke around the rink for me?"

While she skates, I study every inch of her and think, *Don't be overly critical, Madz. You're not Nathan, and this girl will never compete in a qualifying competition.* I wonder where to begin. She's a technical disaster. The judges for her pre-tests must have been lenient. They may have considered how difficult it must have been for her to test in worn-out skates with inadequate ankle support.

Switching gears isn't easy. I need to coach this girl in such a way that I don't kill the joy I see on her face as she skates. After two laps, she closes in and snowplows me—one thing she's good at. Her brother told me she's fourteen. Based on her communication style, I would've guessed she's a tall ten.

I brush the snow off my leg. "You need to straighten up when you skate." I grip her shoulders and pull them back. "Hold your arms up like this." I demonstrate. "And make sure you bend those knees and push off your free leg when you do your crossovers in the corners. Let's go." I demonstrate, then follow her around the rink. I manipulate her shoulders, arms, and hands, correcting her position whenever necessary. Meaning *constantly*.

Next, I watch her skate around the rink on her own.

Better.

I spend the next fifteen minutes going over the proper way to do forward and backward crossovers. Following her around the rink, I coach her: "Bend those knees and push off with the inside edge. Put that same edge down when you cross over. Step forward on the outside edge. Keep those arms up." She follows through with my directions well. Either her former coaches didn't teach her the basics well enough or she simply needed a reminder.

During the last half hour, I assess her single jumps and her spins. She lands the jumps but slouches during them and sometimes wobbles on the landing. This suggests a weak core and, again, poor ankle support. Her spins travel, loop away from her starting point, meaning they aren't centered. Of course not. She haphazardly whips into them, her arms beating the air.

Nathan would say, "What the hell was that?"

I say, "Good effort, but try this." I demonstrate. "Your turn."

She skates to the center of the rink and tries another spin. I coach her throughout it: "Bend your skating knee going into the spin. Straighten your skating knee while spinning. Press your shoulders down, but keep your arms up. Lower your arms."

Whoops. She falls.

I skate closer to her. "You okay?"

"Yes."

"You lifted your arms too high. Remember to press down on your shoulders as you lift your arms."

She goes into the spin again. This time, her soft expression hardens with determination. Entering the spin, she whips her arms around and falls again.

"Gracie." I signal her to skate to me. "Watch my arms as I enter the spin." I stroke to the center of the ice, turn, back-crossover, and step into the spin. "Watch how steady my arms are as my blade *hooks* the three-turn and my skating leg *straightens* up." Spinning slowly, I say, "Now, watch how the spin stays centered as I pull my arms in and speed up." I twirl a basic one-foot spin, then toe-pick the ice to stop. No need for a fancy finish at this point. I skate back to her. "Your turn."

This is bearable. My feet are on the ice without my having to overly exert myself. I could get into this. Such an easy way to earn money. Such an easy way to pay back her brother.

Gracie's back crossovers scratch the ice as she sets up a spin, but I stop myself from criticizing her. One thing at a time. Her crinkled brow and protruding tongue tell me she's concentrating on my directions, albeit putting herself at risk of biting her tongue off if she falls. I should have had her try the spin from a basic three-turn. Next time I will.

Uh-oh, this is not going to end well. Entering the spin, she whips her arms around again. Anticipating her fall, I cringe.

Ouch.

Along with the arm-whipping, she sprang up too hard and fast on her spinning leg. Which I didn't think was possible for a non-flying spin. And she didn't press down on her shoulders but raised them, probably because she was concentrating on straightening out her spinning-leg knee.

She stands, picks her skating dress out of her butt, and marches over to me with tight lips, a crinkled-up chin, and her inner brows plowing into the bridge of her nose. She stops directly in front of me and screams. "Ahhhhhhhhhhhhhh!"

What. The. Fu—

"Shh!" a girl says as she skates by, performing her program.

Finger over my lips, I shush Gracie as well. So embarrassing. I pull my hood over my head. *Sorry*, I mouth to a coach scowling at me. That pink human siren has ruined my reputation.

Her brother knocks on the plexiglass. "Gracie." He points at her. "Knock it off, or the proctor will kick you off the ice."

"I suck!" she yells to him.

He signals her to meet him at the rink's entrance, which is open and thus free of the plexiglass barrier. As he speaks to her, two women in the bleachers lean toward each other and chatter as they leer at Gracie and her brother.

A moment later, Gracie skates back to me. "I'm sorry," she says. "Even though I'm not really."

I can't.

I skate to her brother. "So badly I want to pay you back ASAP, but what's up with this? I don't do scenes, especially those involving inappropriate screaming. Totally unacceptable, and she told me she's not really sorry."

"Wow, you give up easily, huh? Is that why your parents wouldn't pay for your test? You had a tough day, so you tested out and quit competing?"

Those words flip a switch in me that instaboils my blood. "You'll never know what I put into my skating. Never. So don't think your snark can get to me." He just got less cute. I check the clock, skate to Gracie, and get into character as *coach* to knock off the few minutes we have left of this godforsaken lesson. People are watching, and I'm going to show them Madz Monroe is a professional.

"Watch me," I say to Gracie. I enter a one-foot spin from a three-turn. "Watch my arms. Now watch me bend into the three-turn, hook it, and straighten up." I spin a few rotations. "Now you do it. No big deal. Think of what you saw me do as you do it. No pressure. Just do what you saw me do."

"Stop saying *do* so much," she says. "It's annoying."

I roll my eyes, joining the ranks of everyone else here.

She completes what I asked her to do. When she skates back to me, my hand's in the air, and we high-five. The end-of-session buzzer buzzes. Praise. The. Lord.

"Oh no," she says. "I didn't do my routine."

"We'll go over that next time." I smile and nod to prevent another vocal eruption.

We sit on the bleachers and take off our skates. She struggles to undo her bow's double knot, so I undo it for her.

"How many sessions have you skated this week?" I ask.

"Two," she says, pulling off her skates. "This one and the maneuvers session before it."

"You should loosen your laces more before taking off your skates."

"I know." She wipes her blades dry with a dirty rag.

I hand her a clean one from my stash. "Use this. You should only wipe your blades with clean rags, so make sure to wash them. Also, if you want to get better, you should skate two freestyle sessions a day, at least three times a week." I cover my blades and bag my skates.

Gracie does the same. She hands me the rag.

"Keep it. Better to have a couple."

"I don't have enough money for all those sessions. My brother says we can't go into the poorhouse for skating."

Her comment sparks my curiosity, again, over why he, instead of his parents, worries about the skating budget. Their financial situation highlights the difference between Super-Edge skaters and regular skaters. SuperEdge skaters have parents who would go into the poorhouse for their kids' skating. I've heard of parents taking out second mortgages to pay for the kind of training I've gotten. Even so, most parents there have money, and they hand it out like candy on Halloween. Membership fee, coaching fee, choreographer's fee, off-ice training fee, Pilates fee—"Here you go, take it all, just make sure my kid wins something."

"Your brother says you passed your pre-tests. Have you started working on the next ones?"

She's looking over my head at him.

"*Hel-lo*, Gracie," I say, waving my hand. "Did you hear my question?"

"Yeah," she says, still staring over my head. "I know the maneuvers routine but have trouble holding my edges." Her gaze returns to the general vicinity of me. "My old coach cut my freestyle music and put together a program, but I haven't practiced it much. I can't remember all of it."

"Did she give you a list of all the elements you need for the freestyle test?"

"No."

"I'll print one out so you can practice them when I'm not with you. Can you text me a file of your music?"

"I will," her brother says, walking toward me.

"I can do it." Gracie's thumbs go to work. "Here." She passes me her phone. "Put your name and number in my contacts." As I do it, she says, "The song is 'This Is Me' from *The Greatest Showman*. Did you ever see that movie? You should see how big the elephants are. Can you come to my house and watch it?"

"Gracie," her brother says. He shakes his head and says to me, "Sorry."

My phone pings in receipt of her music file.

"The truth is, Gracie"—I look her in the eye—"I love that movie. It's a forever classic." She smiles. "But I can't come over any time soon. I have lots of things going on." I glance at her brother. He's gawking at some chick who's inappropriately dressed for the rink. "Someone should've alerted her to the hazards of wearing six-inch heels to a rink."

"She's not here to skate," he says to me. "Hey," he says to her.

She hugs him. "Hey, Cowboy."

Ugh, give me a break. She eyes me up and down, a short process given that I'm sitting.

"Hi, I'm Madz," I say to her.

She smirks. "Madz?"

"Madelyn," Gracie's brother says.

"Madz," I say. "But don't worry. I'm sure you won't be in a position to have to say it again." I shrug and flash her a fake smile. "Lucky you."

Gracie points to the girl. "You made a face when you heard the name *Madz*. That was rude."

Pure honesty. Quite refreshing. Maybe I'll let the screaming incident slide.

The rude chick, whose name I don't know because she didn't reciprocate the introduction, takes my landscaper's arm and pulls him toward the exit. If he likes a girl who'd smirk at the sound of a new acquaintance's name, I'm glad I didn't take him up on his movie offers. Hmph.

Gracie zips her bag. "Wait, Will!"

Bingo. *Will*. Come to think of it, my father called Will by name before. As Mom pulled into the driveway, Dad realized he'd forgotten their anniversary. He grabbed a vase from the pantry and hollered out to Will, who was working in the yard, "Will, will you cut me enough hydrangeas to fill this?" I thought the double "will" was a nervous stutter resulting from the major time crunch Dad was on.

"Wait up, Gracie," I say. "You did a good job. You tried really hard, and you ended the session with a well-done spin. That's something to be proud of, okay?"

"Okay," she says, craning her neck, looking in Will's direction.

"Text me the days you're skating again. Other than a doctor appointment, my schedule's open."

"Okay, bye." She scurries to Will, interrupting his tête-à-tête with Heels the Rude One.

When I stand, blood whooshes from my head. I sit, take a deep breath, and rest my head in my hands. In the darkness, I hear the pitter-patter of feet. Judging from the voice, they're Gracie's.

"Are you sick? Do you need a ginger ale? I have five dollars. I'll get you one."

Will's voice: "C'mon, Gracie."

Without looking up, I give her the thumbs-up. "I'm fine, thanks, Gracie. Go ahead." As the blood returns to my head and the dark veil lifts from my vision, a wave of relief washes over me. I won't be drawing more attention to myself by passing out.

Gracie can't be too bad of a girl; she cared enough to check on me. I think I get why she got agitated on the ice. She wasn't asking for much. All she wanted was a basic spin, the equivalent of my wanting a double axel yesterday. I totally wanted to scream, "I suck!" at the top of my lungs for screwing up that jump.

SIX

Doctor Weston hangs his stethoscope around his neck. "How long have you had the ache in your chest?"

"About a month. It comes and goes."

He pats my neck with his fingertips, presses into my armpits, then pulls the foot of the exam table out. I lie on my back. I'm not in the mood to laugh, yet I have to force myself not to as he prods my abdomen. I contract my abs and bite my lips, wishing I weren't so ticklish. My wish is granted seconds later.

"Relax your muscles, Madz." He presses deep beneath my left ribcage, triggering an urge to whack him.

You're not kneading bread, dude. That's my spleen you're about to rupture. His previous lymph-node fishing expeditions were picnics compared to this excavation.

"Have you had night sweats?" he asks.

"No, but my mother gets hot flashes. Should we be concerned?" I sit up.

Mom closes her laptop. "We're not here for me," she says.

Dr. Weston smiles. "Your mother's fine." He sanitizes his hands.

Like, I took a shower, guy. You're not gonna get a disease from me.

He sits in front of his computer. "Your spleen isn't enlarged, which is good, but you've lost ten pounds since I saw you six months ago. How's your appetite?"

"Good. Sometimes. I guess it's been kind of lousy. Some-times food smells weird and makes me nauseous."

"You've always been that way," Mom says, fanning herself.

"I know, but it's worse."

"As I mentioned a few years ago, you're a super-smeller," Dr. Weston says, his eyes scanning my electronic record. "You don't have the conditions often associated with hyperosmia, so I'm guessing you inherited it. When you smell something nauseating, suck on a mint or a fruit-flavored hard candy."

Some super-smellers can smell illness, walk into a room of strangers and pick out a person with Parkinson's disease. I mainly scent the foul emissions of death. Dead fish. Dead cow meat. Dead chicken. Dead pork. If I'm within fifteen feet of a store's cold-cut section, I gag.

"Jerry, my daughter's weight loss started last year, after I stopped spending my lunch breaks at SuperEdge and mini-mized my time there on Saturdays. Madz had said my 'heli-coptering'"—she finger-quotes the word—"embarrassed her." She turns to me. "See what happens when I'm not there to push you to finish your lunch or eat a snack?"

Ugh. I lie down again. "I have been eating, even when I don't feel like it. I've been losing weight ever since I caught mono." Infectious mononucleosis, to be exact. Its nickname is *the kissing disease*, which leaves little to the imagination as to how I got it.

"After you get your blood drawn," he says, "go to radiology for a chest X-ray. I should have some answers for you by tomorrow afternoon."

"I think I know the answer, Doctor Weston. I'm exhausted because I haven't had a break in training since I had mono last year. My only other break was when I stress-fractured my tibia four years ago."

"Those were long breaks, Madz. You've only skated for ten and a half months since returning from your mono sabbatical, and during that time, you contracted another strep throat. You had a setback. Strengthen yourself to pre-mono condition, and you won't get so tired." She looks up at Dr. Weston. "Isn't that right, Jerry?"

"I'd expect her to tire more quickly after an illness. However, it's been six months since she had strep throat, longer since having mono. She should feel better by now. As you mentioned, Ava, she trained for years without complaints of fatigue. Mono is caused by the Epstein-Barr virus, which can cause chronic fatigue syndrome. Another thing to consider is that Madz's biological parents were Italian and Greek. Is that correct?"

"Don't forget the dash of Irish," I say.

"Yes, to all of the above," Mom says. "We had her DNA checked."

"I'll check her for thalassemia," Dr. Weston says, "a type of anemia Mediterranean people are prone to."

"Good idea, Jerry," Mom says, "but is she okay to skate?"

I sigh, letting my hands slip from my abdomen and plonk onto the exam table.

"I'm concerned about her weight loss and the enlarged lymph node over her collarbone. Madz should take a break until I see her test results," he says.

I glance at Mom. She's rubbing her forehead and shaking her head.

Dr. Weston eyes her. "Relax, Ava. It's only skating."

I spring up from the jolt of that auditory calamity. Mom's and my eyes collide in a mutual mental gasping.

It's only skating, he said.

I can't undo what I know about the sport. Hours of work and bodily treasure go into perfecting one move, and often several moves go into one jump, one spin, or any combination thereof. Time, money, blood, sweat, tears, sprains, contusions, and cracked bones. They're the dues figure skaters pay for a perfectly executed edge, a centered spin so fast it blurs, and a jump whose lift instills a sense of superpower. In the skating world, sports medicine doctors can achieve rock star status thanks to the sport's demanding nature and physical toll.

Therefore, as much as I believe in free speech, "It's only skating" should never be said to someone with major skin in the game.

"YOU'VE NEVER BEEN the same since you got mono," Mom says. Looking into her compact mirror, she blots her freshly painted lips. "I should report that little shit Joao to the board of health . . . ."

As the droner drones on, I open my music app, put my ear pods in, sit back in my seat, and rest my head against the wall. Nothing's more boring than a radiology waiting room.

I agree with Mom's point about Joao triggering my downward spiral. This is how it happened: He'd arrived from out of state months before and was exceptionally handsome. We became friends, and he told me he was gay. He said he'd never kissed anyone on the lips and asked if I could help him practice.

"Sure," I said. I needed practice myself, and let's face it: how often does a girl get to make out with a gorgeous gay guy? This, I thought, was a once-in-a-lifetime chance, a total win-win.

We made out during lunch break for a week. We'd walk across the street and sit by a narrow section of the Charles River, under a big tree in a private spot. Except for the time a goose claimed it and went Rambo on us. That day, we found a remote space farther away from the river, near a public garden. There, after a warm, lingering kiss, he planted his hand on my left boob.

Wow, I must be a really good kisser, I thought. *I'm heterofying a gay guy.*

"They're small," I said as he pressed his fingers into the side and top of it, kind of how Gallagher taps the top of a cake to see if it's fully cooked.

Joao nodded and furrowed his brow as if he were a doctor assessing a patient. "Small but perky. Lindsey's are floppy. She'd benefit from underwire support."

I recoiled and squinted at him. I wasn't his first choice. Slap my ego much? More important, why practice on two girls? Wasn't kissing one challenging enough for him? And why would this gay guy be boob-curious with me after a flopping experience with Lindsey? Maybe my crystal embellishments lured him into it. Or maybe his having four older sisters prompted a fascination for the functionality of bras.

Common logic stirred doubts about Joao's intentions. My suspicion must have been readable because he said, "I kissed Lindsey once, barely a peck. Her breath killed me." He cringed. "It smelled sick. I thought she might have tonsillitis, but she blamed it on her adenoids."

Up to that point, Lindsey hadn't told me about her interlude with Joao. She had, however, discussed her adenoid issues with me. She said they caused the funny nasal sounds she makes when she speaks, tiny little snorts a highly attentive ear can hear.

In Joao's defense, a person didn't have to be a super-smeller like me to detect the pungent scent of her breath, so I believed him. Still, given the premise of our make-out sessions, the boob fascination and passionate kissing perplexed me. Until I found out that prior to his encounters with Lindsey and me, he'd convinced two other girls to help him "practice kissing." Under the same tree and in the same backup remote spot.

I asked my friend Terrence, a real gay guy who was also a gorgeous skater, to ask out Joao. No gay person in his right mind would turn down Terrence.

"He's not beeping under my gaydar," Terrence said. "What if he's a homophobe? He could get angry and try to beat me up."

"I doubt it. His national and SuperEdge memberships would be revoked. He'd be completely shunned." I told him to ask Joao out while I was there. Terrence would feel safe, and I'd have the satisfaction of watching Joao squirm.

Instead of giving Terrence an out-and-out *no*, Joao squeezed my hand and said, "Terrence, buddy, you're a good-looking dude." He looked up at me in a bad-actor sort of way.

"And if Madz here hadn't turned me straight, I would've taken you up on the offer."

With a jerk of my head, I signaled Lindsey and the two other girls Joao had made out with. They scurried to the table and stood by it with their arms crossed, eyes fixed on Joao.

Terrence stood up, said "Good luck, honey" to Joao, and left, marking the end of Joao's make-out scam. Not to mention my days of feeling healthy and rested. My neck glands swelled, and I tested positive for mono *and* strep throat. The former made my spleen swell, forcing me off the ice. Falling could have made the thing rupture.

I returned six weeks later, trained six days a week while steadily losing stamina, and the rest is history. Thanks, Joao, for kicking off my epic descent.

After I get x-rayed, we head to the lab and get my blood drawn. Leaving the hospital, I say, "I'm going to bed as soon as we get home."

Mom sighs.

I'm sure she thinks I'm lazy. "The doctor said I should take a break. Resting is a compulsory element of a break."

"Okay," she says. "But soon we'll see if anything is, in fact, wrong."

I hate when she uses *in fact* mid-sentence. She's parenting a kid, not prosecuting a case.

MOM PULLS INTO THE GARAGE, and I open my eyes. Home at last. My first day of rest was a never-ending to-do list: test, teach, doctor exam, and test, again, at the hospital.

After shutting off the engine, she checks her messages.

"Nathan texted me. He wants me to congratulate you on passing your final skating test."

"Tell him thanks."

She points at me. "*That* was sass." She throws open her door. "You tell him."

You're proud of me, Mom? Thanks. Your support means the world to me. I really missed having you there with me, especially since I was taking my last skating test ever. Oh, you hope I feel better? Thanks. I do too. It sucks being tired all the time, and the mirror scares me these days. My hip bones poke out, and my cheeks sink in. Have you noticed?

When I get to the kitchen, I open the French doors and breathe in the fragrances of spring—grass, flowers, life. "The yard is quiet without Will."

"Who?" Mom says.

"The landscaper," Dad says, reading something on his tablet and chewing his filet mignon. "He's working on a vacant lot, competing in a community landscaping competition." Dad, Mister Nonconversationalist, knows this. While Mom and I were locked inside our own heads, living within the isolated bubble of figure skating, a whole different world bustled beyond the rink walls. Without us.

I wonder if landscaping is as demanding as figure skating. I imagine cut fingers and sunburns are common among the landscaping elite. Hearing about Will's landscaping competition, I've grown a little envious. As much as I've always loved skating (up until now, of course), I've always loved the idea of landscaping. More so, designing landscapes.

There lies the problem. I loved the *idea*. I should be doing it.

I designed the backyard landscape. Dad encouraged me to

after I told him how I envisioned it: a rustic patio before the French doors, lavender by the gazebo, cone-shaped topiary trees on either side of the entrance to the pool area, impatiens along the walkway to the poolhouse, hydrangeas beside the poolhouse, rhododendrons behind it in a back corner of the yard, arborvitae along the fence, and a spiral-shaped topiary tree planted in the space I view from the breakfast nook.

The house phone rings, but we continue eating because why answer the house phone when only scammers and tele-marketers call? I take my plate to the sink.

"I'm going to bed." The house is so silent the words echo. "Good night." I kiss my parents before going upstairs.

SHOWERED AND IN MY PAJAMAS, I plop on my bed and scroll through social media, admiring shots of my friends having fun. At the skating club, they smile in a group selfie in front of the locker-room mirror, the red squiggles of my lipstick rant hardly visible. Lindsey posted a picture of herself and our friend sitting on the beach wall, eating ice cream. The ocean glistens behind them, and the evening sun casts a soft glow on their faces. I comment under the image: *Take me next time* [*smile face with sunglasses*].

My heavy, bobbing eyelids close, only to fling open when Mom sits on the side of my bed.

"That call during supper was Doctor Weston's office. After you went upstairs, Jerry called my cell phone."

"Already?"

"He promised me he'd expedite the process. I might have pressured him a little."

Translation: she pressured him a lot. "Did he tell you my bloodwork's good and I'm just lazy?"

"No." Her voice cracks, and a sob bursts through her flinty facade.

So much for her suck-it-up policy. "You're scaring me, Mom." As a soon-to-be recipient of bad news, I'd prefer it be delivered with a fake smile and a silver lining.

I rein in my fear, figuring a slightly abnormal result could've rattled her. She's worn out from two consecutive days of Madz-induced stress. I hand her a tissue. "If he figured out why my body's falling apart, don't worry. I can handle it. I mean, how bad can it be?"

"You're anemic. Not the Mediterranean kind of anemia."

"I can get my blood count up. At least we have an explanation for why I'm tired. See? Wasn't so ba—"

"And you have a mass in your chest. He saw it on the X-ray."

I press around my boobs, thinking, *Don't tell me Joao affected them too.* "No, I don't." I'm sure it wasn't there last year. Given the concentration on his face when he poked around, Dr. Joao would've picked up on any lumps and alerted me. Then again, the crystals on my dress could have masked a lump.

"It isn't in your breast tissue. It's inside your chest, behind your sternum. Jerry thinks it's related to that swollen gland in your neck." She holds my hand and sighs. "To diagnose the problem, a surgeon will have to biopsy the lump growing over your clavicle."

SEVEN

Spooked by Dr. Weston, Mom didn't pester me for sleeping throughout most of the weekend, for not utilizing every second of the day effectively. In fact, Gallagher brought breakfast to my room this morning. Other than the eerie sense that something's wrong with me, it's a perfect Sunday.

I sit on the edge of the deep end, dipping my feet in the pool. As I search the internet for landscape images, a fleeting chest ache reminds me of the "mass." What more can squeeze into my chest? It's already filled to max capacity—a heart, two lungs, an esophagus. Scary as it is, I'd be relieved if the thing explained the cause of this annoying ache and life-maiming exhaustion.

Before I contracted mono, morning couldn't come soon enough. I looked forward to going to the rink and working on my jumps, spins, footwork—all of it. I couldn't wait to show Nathan what I could do. Back then, I really did love skating, and falls hurt less. If only I could have jarred that energy. I'd open the lid and suck it all in.

Mom sits next to me, rolls up her pants, and dips her feet in the pool. "Yikes, it's cold."

"It's only been open for a week. Like you always said, the sun will eventually warm the winter out of it." I lift my feet out of the water, wiggle my toes, and dunk them again.

"The skating club's having a farewell barbecue for George. He's moving out of state. How about we go for a few minutes? To wish him well."

"You're not embarrassed to face everyone after what I did?"

"I'm over it."

George has worked in the office and checked me into skating sessions since I joined SuperEdge. I should go. It's an outdoor party, so I can always hide in the car if a smell or a general sense of awkwardness gets to me. Best of all, Nathan won't be there. He only socializes with us peons during the club's yearly Awards Night Banquet.

"Dad said he'd go," Mom says. "Can you believe it?"

I don't believe Dad's going for George, someone he's never met. Like Nathan, my father's a hobnobbing minimalist. I believe Dad's going because he's worried, which worries me. My health condition prompted Mom to cry. My gut says it triggered Dad's sudden interest in attending a parking-lot barbecue. As if it's our last chance for a family outing.

I can only conclude the forecast for Tuesday, the day of my biopsy, is cloudy with a chance of cancer.

LINDSEY'S MOTHER tilts her head, holds out her arms, and pouts, miming, *Your mother told me, you poor thing.* I don't even have a diagnosis yet, and she hugs me as if I'm a goner. Does she know something I don't?

Don't obsess, I tell myself. My neck lump and chest mass are either due to a minor problem or a serious one. Period. Nothing can change what they already are.

I break free from Lindsey's mother's clutches, hug George, and wish him well. Lindsey pulls my arm, walking me toward the food table. "My mother told me about the thing in your chest. What is it? Please tell me it's not breast cancer."

"It's not. The doctor thinks it's related to a swollen neck gland. I'm hoping it's just a weird infection antibiotics can get rid of."

Lindsey takes a paper plate from the table. "I heard you coached a screamer at our old rink. Why would you do that to yourself? You're self-sabotaging lately. I'm worried about you." She fills her plate with ribs, potato salad, and a piece of George's "Good Luck" cake.

"Long story, and no need to worry. I'm doing a favor for someone. How did you find out?"

"My old coach. She texted my mother." She hands me a paper plate. "Take a few ribs. I'll eat them." She peers out the corners of her eyes at her mother, who's conversing with my parents. "You're still a vegetarian, right?"

"Sort of. I'm an extremely reluctant carnivore." I'm prone to anemia, so my parents insist I eat red meat once a week. Which guarantees a weekly tug-of-war between my gag reflex and me and a weekly guilt trip over the poor cow sacrificed for the sake of my blood count.

She loads my plate, aka hers, with ribs. "Ooh, I'll try these too." She adds a cookie and a scoop of pasta salad, and the paper plate bends from the weight.

After a brief juggle, I save the food. "Careful, Lindsey, your food's about to flop onto the asphalt."

"Shh, why did you say it was my food?"

"Uh, because it is?"

"Shh. My mother might hear. I don't want a freaking lecture about recommended daily allowances."

"You're skating again. You'll burn it off." *Yech*, this meat stinks. I hand her the plate. "Take this. The ribs. I can't . . ."

"I'll be right back." She puts her plate on a table, returns, and takes the reeking plate from me.

Will texts me: *My sister is skating. Where are you?*

This kid can't be serious. We made a deal I'd teach his sister, not be at his beck and call. I text him where I am and remind him we didn't schedule a lesson for Gracie today. Then I get an idea.

I call Will and say, "I can give her an off-ice lesson tonight at my house. In my gym. Does she have any physical limitations I should be aware of?"

"Other than slightly uncoordinated fine motor skills, she has no physical limitations that I'm aware of. I'll text you after she skates and let you know if she'll do it or not."

"Okay, but tell her I can teach her all day long on the ice, but if she doesn't train off of it, she's more at risk of hurting herself and ruining her chances of being a successful skater." By learning a conditioning routine, Gracie can continue to build her strength and stamina even after I fulfill my obligation to her brother. I don't hold a certification, but I've taken enough lessons to earn an honorary doctorate in training.

"She's always refused to work out with me, but okay. I'll tell her it's part of your teaching program. Gotta go. Bye."

He probably has no idea what I was talking about. Off-ice training isn't necessarily about going to the gym. It's about conditioning the body for skating. This includes exercises for improving balance, flexibility, and strength: Pilates, plyometrics, ballet, stretching, weights, cardio, and more.

My training-session idea is genius. I'll be killing two birds with one stone, knocking off my obligation hours and avoiding the embarrassment of her screaming in front of the other coaches.

"Mmm," Lindsey says, eating pasta salad. "This is freaking delicious. I forget; why do we starve ourselves?"

"We don't. We make nutritious choices, practice calorie awareness, and allow ourselves an occasional treat." *Like the ice cream you enjoyed at the beach without me.*

"You sound like Nathan."

"Did he take you on as a student?"

"Fresh off a back injury? Of course not. At the rate I'm going, I'll be on that freaking waiting list until the day I die. In the meantime, I pay close attention to his students' techniques during jumps, spins, et cetera, and watch his response. If Nathan nods, I imitate what the skater did. If he shakes his head, I listen to what he tells the skater. If I can't hear or he doesn't demonstrate, I watch the skater for technique changes during the next attempt and see how it works out. Kind of like analyzing before-and-after pictures. I learn without having to put up with Nathan's rates or attitude."

"Careful, Lindsey. I think espionage is illegal. I can tell you what he told me if you want to know."

"Yes, I do want to know. But right now all I want to know is this gorgeous rib." She bites into it. "Mmm. Taste the barbecue sauce," she says with a full mouth, waving the rib in front of my face. "It's delicious."

A set of coconut-scented hands creep up from behind me and cover my eyes. "Why do you look like you're going to throw up?" Joao says into my ear. He unblinds me.

"Because you're here," Lindsey says, stomping away.

"Why can't she get over it already?" he says.

"I guess you're a tough guy to get over."

"I am. Aren't I?"

He could pass for Will's younger brother. One big difference, Joao would never let a piece of hair fall out of place. He's the only skater I know who can end a session of spinning and jumping looking the same as when he started. He attributes this to multiple applications of organic hair gel, the origin of the coconut aroma on his hands.

"So," he says, "it hasn't been a week since you quit skating, and you're already teaching?" He points at me. "Don't say you're not. I heard you on the phone, talking to someone about off-ice training." He drops his annoying pointer finger and stares at SuperEdge's newest member as she walks by. He winks at her.

"Really? She's, like, twelve."

"She's a petite fifteen. Her mother says she's turning sixteen in the fall. Only a year younger than me. Anyway, where were we? Oh. Can I be honest with you, Madz?"

"Bring it on."

"I'm worried about you. I mean, you loved skating up until last year. I can't help but think I had something to do with your leaving."

My phone buzzes with a text from Will: *She said okay.*

Don't give her too much information at once or she'll get frustrated. Her auditory processing trips up. And start her off slowly. She never worked out before.

Gracie's text pops up next: *This stupid lesson of yours better be fun. I hate working out.*

Joao waves his hand between my phone and me. "Earth to Madz."

Rude. "I hate to break the news to you, but no, you were not a factor in my leaving here." He piles ribs onto a plate, drowning the pleasant coconut aroma and heightening my sense of urgency to run. "I have to go."

I scurry to my car to escape the death smell and the urge to rant about his contribution to my physical downfall.

In the car, the heat sinks into my skin, slow-roasting me like a rotisserie chicken. Mom hops in, starts the car, and turns on the AC. She hands me a bottle of water.

"Drink. My God, it's hot in here. It's a good thing I checked on you."

Dad gets in the back seat. "Are we done mingling?"

"Yeah, let's go." I expect an argument but don't get one. As we drive off, Joao waves to me, but Lindsey's preoccupied. She's sitting at a picnic table, giggling with fellow SuperEdge skaters. To her, I guess I'm just a vehicle for extra servings of food.

It's been three days since I quit skating. I was a fixture here. You'd think one of my skating "friends" would have come to the car and said hi—or goodbye. Whatever. Who would have thought Joao would be the most concerned about my motivation for leaving this place?

"Why didn't you sit with your friends?" Mom says.

"They're doing fine without me."

"They're probably afraid to associate with you. God forbid Nathan sees them talking to someone who walked out on one of his lessons."

What she said would be inappropriate if it weren't true. They witnessed me walk out on my lesson with him. Half of them have him as a coach; the other half want him as a coach. No way the latter half will stay on his waiting list if they nuzzle up to me.

"I think you should talk to a psychologist," Mom says. "Someone nonjudgmental, who's an expert in helping teenagers work through difficult situations and emotions."

Can't a girl feel like crap, avoid people, and rest without bringing a coach into the equation? That's what a psychologist is, an emotion coach. Until today, I handled my departure from skating better than Mom. And she's the one who cried over my abnormal X-ray.

"I'm good, thank you." The hardest thing I face is the unknown, a "difficult situation" talking won't fix.

EIGHT

The security monitor in the kitchen shows Will and Gracie hopping out of Will's pickup truck and heading to our front door. "Who are these people?" Mom says, peering out the window. Gallagher stands beside her, doing the same. The doorbell rings, and Mom runs to the wine refrigerator. She opens a bottle of Pinot Grigio while I greet our guests at the door.

"Are you coming in?" I ask Will, hoping to hear more about this landscape competition he participated in.

"Can't, thank you. I have to do something."

"Take your time," Gracie says.

I suspect she's not aware her brother "contracted" me for a specific amount of time. Ugh, I wonder if she even knows about the deal. If not, how am I supposed to tell her in another week that I'm done giving her lessons? I don't have a psych degree, and this girl can read a situation. A fake smile won't lessen the blow of this bad news, and with her reputation and limited finances, there's no silver lining to her losing me as a coach.

Will better have planned for the grand finale of our deal, Gracie's last lesson. It would be a travesty if he led his sister to believe I'd be her permanent coach.

IN THE GYM WITH GRACIE, I avoid lengthy explanations and teach her warm-ups by demonstrating—works for her learning style. She follows my moves on the agility ladder and lunges with me in various directions during plyometric exercises. She's huffing and puffing, so I limit her to one set of each. Works well for me because I'm huffing and puffing myself.

"If you do these warm-ups regularly," I say, "they'll get easier." To convince her, I force myself not to pant. "I usually do three sets of each." I sit, relieved to have an excuse to do so. "Your sneaker's untied. Lace up before we move on."

She crouches over her sneaker, brow crinkled and tongue peeking out as she slowly goes through the motions of tying. From an onlooker's standpoint, it's a real nail-biter, a struggle to watch. Similar to her attempt at undoing the double knot in her skate laces. The good news, neither this nor the double-knot debacle at the rink psyched her out to the point of screaming, and she succeeds in tying her sneaker. Loosely.

I tighten the bow for her, and we move on to the routine my parents paid an abundance of hundreds to ingrain into my being. To improve her balance and strengthen her core, we play catch with a medicine ball while balancing on one foot. We also do plank pushups. I have her do them on her knees, a modified version for beginners. She struggles through a few banana rolls, and then we jump rope.

Finally, we go through the motions of jumps she performs on the ice. The first three we tackle are the waltz jump, Salchow, and toe loop. She gathers momentum for each by side-hopping. Similar to how she did them on the ice, she slouches during the jumps. Upon landing, she swings her arms way up, then down—a giant flap—indicating she has no idea where they must be and why. Same with her legs. During her loop, flip, and Lutz, she whips her arms around, spinning rather than going up and pulling in. Her legs separate in the air rather than stay together as they should.

The hour's up in a flash. Raining sweat, she exerted herself more during this lesson than the on-ice one, yet she never screamed. "You did a great job, Gracie."

"You tried to kill me." She wipes her forehead with the back of her hand.

As she gulps her water, I show her a printout of the exercise routine. "You need to go through this warm-up a few times a week whether I'm around or not. The least you should do before skating is jump rope and stretch." I take her to the ballet bar and show her stretches before we go.

Gracie hugs me. "You're nice to let me come here and to teach me all of this stuff."

"You might not like me much tomorrow," I say. "Other than stretching, give your body a break tomorrow and do something fun."

"This was fun." She looks at her phone. "Will's here."

We scurry upstairs, and I walk her to the front porch.

"When can you coach me on the ice again?" she asks, her eyes wide as she awaits my answer.

Will honks the horn, putting the pressure on. I wave to him and say to Gracie, "Let me check my schedule."

I lock the front door and catch a glimpse of Mom. In the kitchen, she sits at the granite island, sniffling, blotting her nose, a half-empty bottle of wine in front of her. Gallagher looks at her and shakes his head.

Caught him. He "broke character," beyond his occasional *Ha!,* during working hours. I'm not the only one who thinks Mom's being overly dramatic.

I grab a spoon from the utensil drawer, take a yogurt and a bin of blueberries from the fridge, and sit at the table.

"You trained with Harvard-bound, elite skaters at the best skating club in Massachusetts, and you're hanging out with the landscaper's little sister. Who skates at what, pre-test level?"

"She likes to skate. I figured I'd teach her off-ice conditioning."

"I realize you have a legitimate health issue, Madz, but if you're *sooo* tired and, in your words, 'done' with skating, how did you drum up the energy to train her?"

I've avoided telling her about Will's donation to the Madz Monroe Skating Test Foundation. She'll be pissed.

"If you plan to coach," she says, "you should invest your time and sweat in someone with a higher potential for success. Someone who'll represent you better."

Everything's a competition with her. "I represent myself, Mom. And Gracie? She strives to succeed, but will her definition of success match yours or anyone else's?"

I'm not in the mood for a philosophical discussion about success, and by withholding the truth from Mom, I'm restless in my own skin. I'd rather be honest, weather the fallout, and be done with it.

"That said, I'm not going to lie to you." *The wine will ease the blow*, I tell myself. I pour more into her glass. "Gracie, as I've told you, is Will's sister. The landscaper has a name, Mom, and it's Will. Do you hear me?"

"I'm listening." She puts down her glass. I try to pour the last of the bottle into the goblet, but she covers the rim with her hand.

"Don't be mad, okay?"

"Go on," she says.

"He gave me money for my test. And practice ice. Plus ten extra dollars for unplanned expenses. I used it for gas."

"How much did he give you altogether?"

"One hundred and fifty dollars."

Her lips tighten into a thin line.

I push forward. "In return, I committed to giving Gracie three one-hour lessons."

Mom's eyes widen.

"I only have one hour left. One hour, then I owe Will nothing."

She opens her purse. "Give him the whole thing." She slides 150 in cash to me.

Blood rushes to my head, and my stomach churns with the queasiness of regret. I shouldn't have told her. I want to pay Will in full—the sooner, the better—but these uneasy symptoms warn me that taking her money isn't the right thing to do.

"I don't need it," I tell her. "I don't owe him this much anymore."

"I refuse to be indebted to my teenage landscaper." She rests her face in her hands. "Why is this happening?"

"You're not indebted to the landscaper. I am. I made a deal with him and won't renege on it. You're a lawyer. You, of all people, should encourage me to follow through with a verbal contract. This one doesn't just involve money. It involves an actual human, his sister, who's counting on me. *Jeez.*"

"You've embarrassed the family. We have enough money. We don't need to borrow anyone else's."

"I didn't have access to your money, remember? You didn't want me testing."

If I had paid back Will in full, she'd still mull over my having borrowed money from him. The aversion stems from her childhood. Growing up, her parents fought a lot over money. She told me more than once that her father was "always borrowing from Peter to pay Paul." Before I knew it was a mere expression, I wondered if Peter and Paul had ever figured out what was going on.

The following words won't help my loan case. I say them, anyway, to support the notion I borrowed responsibly, the opposite of what her father did. "I gave Gracie a skating lesson the day I took my test. Today's off-ice lesson makes two hours. One more hour, and I'm done paying back Will. I'll save better from now on, and we'll never have to have this conversation again. Lesson learned. Case closed."

Her thumbs tap away on her cell phone. I guess I wasted my breath.

"Who are you texting?"

Her thumbs stop moving. She removes her readers and smacks them on the counter. "Done," she says with a smirk.

"What?"

"I fired that little shit. I transferred two hundred and fifty dollars to his direct-pay app. It covers what you borrowed and what I owe him for yard work."

"First of all, he's not a little shit. He's six feet and ripped, has his own business, and will be a senior in high school in the fall. Second of all, I . . . I made a deal. I did. And you . . . you embarrassed me by saying that to him. I don't like you." Monster tears storm down my face.

"I didn't hire him to invade my life."

F-ed up, served hot on a silver platter. "So wrong, and you know it. You're acting like the Wicked Witch." Gallagher must agree. He's shaking his head at her again. I race to my room, throw myself on my bed, and cry myself to sleep.

NINE

A mourning bird coos, waking me up. I sweep my fingers across the bedside table and tap the remote control. The curtains open, the shades lift, and the sun slips in and pries my eyes open. My left leg slips off the side of the bed, sending a wake-up call to the rest of my body.

I stare at the ceiling. *What am I getting up for?* I don't have to race to the rink, an off-ice class, or my skate-sharpening guy. I completed my spring-semester online classes. And I don't want to face my mother. I'm fuming over her firing Will, and she had the nerve to work from home today.

I'm in trouble if hibernating in my room is the best I can do on a sunny first-of-June morning. It's the first Monday of my post-skating life, and I have no game plan other than to dodge Mom. I'm in foreign territory.

My situation reminds me of a former figure-skating champion I read about. She went into a depression after her body reached its wear-and-tear limit at twenty, forcing her into retirement. Outside the skating world, she didn't know her purpose in life. Up to that point, her whole identity had been attached to the sport.

She pulled herself out of her depression by earning a doctorate in alternative medicine and writing books about her specialty, but she never again set foot in a rink. After all those years of training.

What. Was. It. All. For? The money, the bruises, the pressure over landing jumps and winning.

Maybe someday I'll find the answer to that question.

Okay. I'm on vacation in foreign territory. Vacations are supposed to be fun. They're fun because . . .

It's fun to be free. Of time constraints. Of pressure to perform. Of pain.

I could go to the beach and dip my feet into the ocean. Which is loaded with pee. Fish pee and people pee. Yuck. The upside to fish pee is the phosphorous it contains. Coral reefs depend on it. I covered the topic in a science report I called "Necessary Evils of the Ocean."

The beach won't be fun without my friends. It's 8 a.m. Whether in school or at SuperEdge, all are busy adhering to their schedules with warrior precision. While their parents maintain a sense of pride, mine must deal with a rogue whose life is on hold.

I can't wait to get this biopsy done tomorrow and treat whatever's wrong with me. *Nothing to do* feels wrong.

I decide on a practical approach: I broke a routine; therefore, I need a new routine. To figure it out, I'll have to familiarize myself with this new terrain. The weather is warm, so I'll put on my sneakers and . . . go for a walk.

There. I made my first time-management decision as a free woman.

My right leg slips off the bed and dangles with the left. I close my eyes, waiting for my upper half to connect with my lower half. Mom's angry face pops into my head. She was so hateful last night. I text Will: *I'm sorry. I'll talk to my father. He likes you.*

I push myself up and sit because nothing will happen unless I make something happen. "Why am I treating going for a walk as a necessary evil?" It's nothing compared to what I did at SuperEdge.

Will texts me back: *Not necessary. BTW, I told Gracie you can't give her lessons anymore. I sent your mother's money back to her, minus what she owes me for yard work, but consider us square anyway.*

Collapsing backward onto the bed, I prepare for a good cry. *Why?* We're not going out. I barely know him or his sister. I paid back two-thirds of what I owed him. He's the one who chose not to take Mom's money or my final lesson.

None of those excuses take away the dis-ease plaguing me over the gross injustice Mom inflicted upon Will. How could she be capable of such evil? I wish I could erase this mortification from my memory bank.

Defying my anger, I yawn, then yawn again.

Three hours later, I wake up with an achy lower back, my legs still dangling over the side of the bed. I stand, touch my toes, and hang there a moment.

My muscles loosen more under a hot shower, relieving my backache, but the steam worsens the fog inside my head. I cool the water to wake myself up.

UNLEASHED FROM THE binding fibers of lycra, my skin adjusts to the easy, breezy freedom of shorts and a cotton T-shirt. I tie my sneakers and scurry downstairs. I peek into Dad's office and wave as he speaks on the phone. He usually does office work here after making his morning rounds on construction sites.

I head to the front door.

"Breakfast first," Gallagher says.

"No, thanks. My appetite's on strike. Maybe a walk will convince it to get back to work—ha ha."

He shakes his head. One of his jobs is making sure I eat breakfast.

I stop at the door. With my parents in their offices and me on my way out, Gallagher might get lonely. "Would you like to come with me?" I ask him.

"Don't wanna slow ya down, love."

"I assure you that won't be a problem. I've aged a hundred years the past few months."

He waves me off, and I head out the front door, down the concrete steps, down the stone-paved walkway, onto the tree-lined sidewalk. Cruising along, I reintroduce myself to my Massachusetts niche.

The last time I walked through the neighborhood, Mom came with me. It happened six years ago on a Sunday morning, the day before I dedicated my entire life to my SuperEdge training. People live in these houses I pass, and I don't know them. I've lived here my whole life, practically, and I don't know my neighbors. The only kids I know from my city are the few I went to private school with before homeschooling.

However, the deeper I delved into figure skating, the further we grew apart.

My lack of neighborly contact doesn't validate the home-school-lack-of-socialization spiel. I met people from across the globe during competitions and while training. I socialized almost daily at SuperEdge and attended its monthly dinners with my friends. Entertainment included musicians, magicians, and in March, Irish step dancers. On the flip side, there was the Joao thing. Where did that get me? Where did socializing, sort of, with Will and Gracie get me?

Socialization is overrated.

A lawn mower moans in the distance, out of view. If it's Will, he's invisible like everyone else in this neighborhood. Craning my neck, I search for his truck.

The mower moans louder, the smell of freshly cut grass grows stronger, as I approach a large white-brick house. It's similar to mine, except mine's made of white-washed red brick, and this one sits on a corner lot and has a lot more adornments, like the fountain front-yard center.

What's this? A weed sticks out of the lawn like a mangy cowlick. I pull it.

Mom thinks the fountain is gaudy, but it's not. Two cherubs hold up a bowl rimmed with lion heads, complementing the lions on either side of the doorway. The plant grouping bothers me. It creates a sense of disorder, a possible reason why Mom perceives the fountain as gaudy.

More weeds. I pull them because I hate them.

Hanging out on the sidewalk, analyzing landscapes, pulling out someone else's weeds? I don't see anything wrong with it. But I'm aware spectators of my life might think I need to get one. I turn the corner, and there it is: Will's pickup truck. It's parked in the driveway of the corner-lot house, partially hidden behind an arborvitae wall.

He emerges from the backyard, pushing his lawn mower. I speed-walk to my house, my arms chugging me along—back and forth, back and forth—like I'm a human locomotive with weeds stuck in its main crank pin. Channeling the Little Engine That Could, I steam up my walkway and front steps, screeching to a halt at the front door. Gallagher opens it before my hand reaches the knob.

Panting in the doorway, I try to catch my breath.

"I see the walk put a bounce in your step." He takes the weeds and guides me to the sink. As I wash my hands, he clears his throat and shifts his eyes toward the breakfast nook. Where Gracie's sitting. "Why don't you ask your company whether or not she'd like to have breakfast with you?" He steps closer to me and whispers, "I found her by the spiral topiary tree."

I approach Gracie, who's looking out the window. This wouldn't be so awkward if Will hadn't texted me what he did. I doubt he'd be okay with her being here. I'm not sure I'm okay with it. Ugh, I hope Mom stays in her office. She's mad enough at Will. Gracie's impromptu visit might add kerosene to the fire.

My deal with Will may have been a deal with the devil, in the form of a fourteen-year-old stalker.

"I wish we had a yard so Will could make me one of those." Gracie presses her index finger against the window, pointing at the spiral-designed topiary tree. "I like the way the leaves swirl up the tree."

I've gazed at the same tree, thinking the same thing. Maybe she's not a stalker. If she were, she'd be more focused on me than a topiary. "Your brother's an artist, and trees are his canvas. Those swirls are called a spiral design."

"They remind me of spins, not spirals."

"Me too. I brought up that point to my skating teacher. I asked him, 'Why is a spiral called a spiral if I'm not spinning around when I'm doing it?' He said if I held on to the edge I did my spiral on and didn't stop, my blade would eventually carve smaller and smaller curves in the ice, forming a spiral pattern."

"Like the spirals Will carves, only his ride up trees."

"Yup."

"He's an artist with pictures too. He can draw anything. And he's an artist with wood. He likes to build things. He made a dollhouse for me one year for Christmas."

Those words pull my heartstrings like a Mac truck. He's an artist *and* a sweet brother. My muscular, snarky landscaper is sensitive. I feel worse than ever over how Mom treated him.

"Wow, is there anything he can't do?"

Gracie stares out the window. Her attention soon turns to Gallagher, who loads the table with food—eggs, waffles, maple syrup, and a bowl of strawberries and blueberries. "Would you like apple or orange juice, lass?" he asks while handing me my OJ.

When I first taught Gracie at the rink, she claimed Will said they couldn't go into the poorhouse for her skating. When I made the deal with Will, he said he'd dropped Gracie's coach because she charged too much for his budget. Will navigates the figure-skating circuit for her. He even finagled a teaching deal with me. The brothers of skaters I know don't involve themselves in their siblings' skating. Where are Will and Gracie's parents?

She settles into her seat. "This is like a restaurant." She tilts her head up to Gallagher. "I want what Madz has, please." She says to me, "Is he your grandfather?"

"No, but he's like one. He's a close family friend."

"Oh. And he comes over to feed you? Did you invite him, or did he just show up like I did?"

"Ha!" Gallagher bursts out as he washes the waffle maker.

"Kind of a long story. Why are you here? Do your parents know? Does Will know? Aren't you supposed to be in school?" It's like Gallagher and I are caring for a stray puppy.

"Kind of a long story." She gnaws her lip and furrows her brow. "If you're not skating or coaching anymore, what will you do? Are you gonna be lazy now? Will says if we're not studying or working, we're lazy."

"I think I'm entitled to a few lazy days after six years of training at SuperEdge." As my eyes follow the lines of the spiral topiary, I see myself swirling through my former rigorous routine.

Also looking at the tree, Gracie says, "You skated. You didn't work."

She did *not* just say that. Peering at her, I give her a piece of my mind. "Number one. I did have an official regular job. I taught group lessons and did substitute coaching." I burned those bridges when I walked out on Nathan. "Are you listening to me, Gracie?"

Still staring outside, she says, "Yeah."

"Number two. Skating itself—all the training, off the ice and on—was a job. No one can tell me it wasn't." For a stray puppy, she's very opinionated.

I dig into my eggs because *protein*. When eating's a matter of survival, not joy, you prioritize nutrition over revulsion.

"Gallagher, did you do something different to the eggs? They smell extra eggy."

"No, love. I made them as usual. Make sure you fill up. You're eating light the rest of the day, and no breakfast tomorrow."

Through a mouthful of waffles, Gracie says, "Why can't you eat breakfast tomorrow?"

"I have this thing to do, and if I eat before it, my stomach will get upset."

She swallows a gulp of juice. "What thing?"

"Just a stupid thing I don't want to talk about." When I had mono, my neck glands were three times bigger than the lump I'm getting biopsied tomorrow. Gallagher thinks my gland has a "fever," but I've never heard of such a thing and can't imagine how a gland fever causes a chest mass.

I pinch my nose and stuff a bite of eggs into my mouth.

Gracie stares at me. "You're weird."

"I know."

She spoons berries onto my plate. "These will freshen your palate."

"Thank you, Miss Fancy Shmancy." I pop one into my mouth. She's right; they do.

My phone buzzes.

"No phone at the table," Gracie says.

I show her my phone. "It's your brother."

She waves her hands. "Don't tell him I'm here."

He asks me if she's here.

"Yes, she is."

"She wasn't supposed to leave the truck," he says. "I only planned to work at your neighbor's for a half hour."

"She's eating. Can she stay a while?"

"Put me on speaker so she can hear me," he says.

On and on and on he goes, complaining about her not listening to him and him having a ton of errands to do. I roll my eyes and Gracie giggles. "If she doesn't come with me now, Madz, I can't pick her up for another two hours."

Gracie perks up. "Okay," she says into my phone. "Okay, Will."

"Two hours is okay," I say.

The call ends, and Gallagher's eyes ping-pong from me to a calmer Gracie.

"Thank you for letting me stay," she says.

"You're welcome." Hmm, in addition to everything else Will does for his sister, he minds her. While he's working. Assuming Gracie's parents work, I remind myself not all working parents have a butler. Besides, Gracie is fourteen, and in spite of her cognitive and, possibly, emotional issues, she's sharp. If a sketch tried to take advantage of her, I think she'd give him a run for his money.

Will texts: *Two hours really ok?*

"Why can't you teach me anymore?" Gracie says. "Is it because I yelled?"

Thanks, Will. I text him *Yeah*, place my phone on the table, and give Gracie my full attention. "Full disclosure, I didn't like the yelling. At all. But that's not why." I should teach her. What else am I going to do with my time?

As I finish my berries, Gracie stares at me.

"I can give you a few more lessons," I say. "It's just—"

"You already paid my brother back."

"No." She knows about the deal, and she's not hurt. One less thing to worry about.

"I'm not stupid. You already paid my brother back, and I

yelled during my lesson. Why would you teach me if you don't have to?"

"I didn't pay him back. I owe him—I mean you—one more hour. But I don't care about the deal. I'll give you as many hours as I can." *Did I just say that? Hel-lo, Madz, you're digging your grave deeper.* "It might not be much. I need a real job."

"How is coaching me not a real job?"

Coaching her is a real job. Unfortunately, once I'm past the hour I owe Will, I'll be coaching her for free. How shallow will I sound if I tell her I need a money-paying job, preferably outside of a rink? "It is a real job. I just have a way of complicating things."

"You say you'll teach me again, but Will says you can't teach me anymore. Was he lying?" She puts her fork down, frowns, twirls her hair between her fingers, then chews on the end of the clump. She twists in her seat and stares at the topiary tree again.

"I wouldn't say he lied. I think he might've gotten the wrong impression from something my mother did. She was mad at me. It's a long story. Anyway, I'll give you another lesson when I can. I have a few things coming up." Like having my neck cut open.

Still staring out the window, she asks, "What's the trick?"

"Trick to what?" I say.

"Doing a spiral. I can do one straight down the ice, but . . ." She untwists and faces me. "When I try to do it on an edge, like I need to do for my test, I always fall off of it."

"Shoulders back, chin up, no hunching over." I get up from the table and demonstrate. "Like this. If you're on a left outside edge, hold your left arm up in front and right arm back, just as you would while holding an edge in a regular, upright position."

She hops out of her seat and tries to copy me.

"You're hunching. Arch your back. Pull your right shoulder back." I grip her arm and gently pull it up and back. "Point your toe like this." I position her foot.

"Ow, I'm not made of rubber."

I place my fingers under her chin. "Chin up."

"It's hard."

"Not if you practice. Just remember to keep your blades sharp and your arms where they need to be. That will help you steer your edge. Didn't your former coach tell you those things?"

"Yeah, but I forgot, and since she dropped me, I had no one to remind me."

"I'll remind you when we're on the ice again. Until then, watch an internet video to refresh your memory. And don't forget. Stretch every day, and do your strength training at least a few times a week. Okay?"

My parents peek around a wall and stare like two scientists monitoring their study subjects.

I lead Gracie downstairs to the gym and run through her warm-up routine. She remembers every detail. I teach her ballet-barre warm-ups for spirals and then lead her to the tread-mill. As she walks, I stand beside her, worried if her coordination will improve enough for her to master the required elements for her next round of tests.

"What are your skating goals?" I ask her. "Like, do you just skate for fun?" Please say yes.

She giggles. "That's why everybody skates."

"I mean, how many tests do you plan to take? Do you plan

on competing?" Test level determines competition level, whether the skater competes individually, in pairs, ice dance, precision skating, or ice theater. Some people who test don't compete. Others compete locally in non-qualifying competitions.

"Uh, yes, I plan on competing. My last coach told me about the Special Olympics. I told her I could skate in regular competitions if I had a competition dress and a regular coach."

"I told your brother you can borrow my dresses. Follow me." I take her to another room on the same floor, my skating "closet." I open the door. "Gallagher nicknamed this room Madz's Hall of Fame. I keep all of my skating stuff in here."

Gracie studies my memorabilia wall. It holds pictures, medals, and platters from local, sectional, and national competitions; pins I got for passing tests, and a wall-length shelf of trophies from competitions as far back as before SuperEdge. One is from my first, when I was five. I won because I was the only contestant.

Another wall is devoted to ice-skate-wearing stuffed animals and skating-themed figurines I've collected over the years. I open a closet. "Test dresses are on the left side; competition dresses, the right. If you ever need one, you're welcome to take your pick."

Gracie's jaw drops. "Wow." A big smile lights up her face.

"Competing is a big commitment, not just for you but for your coach." Not sure if she hears me. Swarovski seems to have cast a spell on her. "Are you listening, Gracie? Look at me." I tap her shoulder, grabbing her attention. "I wish I could help you more with coaching, but I can't. I can give you a lesson here and there, but competitions? I retired from competitive skating. In fact, I retired from skating, period."

Her chest rises and falls with increasing intensity. "What does 'retired from skating, period' mean?"

"It's when you decide to stop skating. Forever." Saying the words out loud, I don't believe them. *Forever* is drastic. Skating for fun? Likely. Coaching? Not out of the question. It's a better way to earn money than making deals with my landscaper. However, I have to fix my broken body first, a subject too complicated to get into with her.

Huffing and puffing through her teeth, Gracie glares at me. "All of this"—she throws her arms out—"and you quit. You *quit* skating. You"—her cheeks flush; her head shakes—"you can't quit skating!"

She's hyperventilating. Sort of. Her hands aren't cramping up like Lindsey's did when she fell and hurt her back during her skating test. Although Gracie's breaths have a gasping quality, they're slower and more controlled than Lindsey's were.

"Gracie, stop. Shh. Gracie, shh." She pushes my hand away when I reach for her shoulder. "I had good reasons. I was wrong for saying forever. I'm giving you a lesson, remember?"

"Madz. Is everything okay down here?" My eyes cling to Mom's as Gracie sits on the floor and cries.

"How can you quit skating? You're too good," Gracie says, waving her hand at my wall of medals. "If I could skate like you, I would win a gold medal. I would jump and spin and do tricky maneuvers like I see on TV. I would stay on the ice forever." She looks up at me, tears welling, pink blotches spattered across her face. "It's not fair."

Mom's chin quivers, and she drops her head. Her sadness over my leaving skating goes deeper than my inability or unwillingness to follow through with her plan. Before she was the prosperous and prominent Ava Monroe, Mom was

Ava Hood, whose parents, like Gracie's, couldn't afford lessons.

Money could have helped Mom reach her skating goals. Unfortunately, it will take more than cash to help Gracie accomplish hers. Despite her keen memory, sharp observation skills, and ability to express herself, Gracie's condition seems to have given her weaker and less-coordinated muscles. I don't think she could ever snap into a double or triple, even if she had constant access to the best coaches and training.

So yeah, now I feel like crap. Safe to say we all do down here in Madz's Hall of Fame.

TEN

racie skips to Will's truck. I assume the bounce in her step came from my promise to give her at least three more lessons and a possible connection with a new, affordable coach. Who, unlike me, isn't retired. The coach promise complicates matters. The best one for her would have experience training Special Olympians, and my contacts are limited.

Translation: I need to humble myself and text Nathan. He's the person my research led me to. Destiny has implanted him in my life like the dandelions in my backyard. I weed him out of my life, and he pops back up.

"Hey," I say to Will. He avoids eye contact.

"Hey, Madz. Gracie, buckle up. We have work to do."

"You're busy, huh?" I say.

"That's an understatement."

Here goes nothing: "If you need extra help, I'm looking for a job." Mom shouldn't disown me for working with him. It's the opposite of borrowing.

Will nods and grins, then his grin twists into a sarcastic smirk. "I do need help. In fact, I have six more jobs to do today. The question is, are you willing to get your hands dirty?" He cocks his head.

I expected sarcasm from him, second-hand punishment for Mom's shenanigans. "I'll be right back."

I run into the house, pull my ponytail through the back of a pink baseball cap, and grab my gardening gloves and three bottles of water. The job offer is like a shot of caffeine, jolting my body out of its weary state.

Mom eyes me as she sits at the table with Dad and Gallagher, who are eating lunch.

"Don't be mad, Mom. I'm working with Will for the rest of the day. It's a paying job. You said I should have one."

Gallagher and Dad fix their eyes on her.

"Be careful," she says to me with a soft smile.

Her days of seeing Will as a "little shit" might be over. Maybe she lightened up because Gracie validated her grief over my leaving skating. Or maybe, just maybe, Mom's relaxed expression, one I can't recall seeing since before our SuperEdge days, means the weight of the rink has also lifted from her.

"FIRST STOP, NORTHERLY HILLS," Will says.

As we pull up to the assisted living complex, an old man waves to us from a bench outside the building. A lady stares at us skeptically as we gather on the lawn. Will orders Gracie and me to weed around the flower beds while he mows the lawn. Then, we rake his clippings after he trims the shrubs.

We finish the job in an hour, but I find more weeds that need pulling. Ugh, they drive me crazy. I grip one and—

"Not those," Will says. "We only pull out the weeds they pay us to pull out, the ones around the flowers. If you want to be a volunteer weed-puller, do it on your own time. We have other jobs to complete." He gives me the same lecture every time we do another job, but I can't resist. Old habits are stubborn beasts.

Throughout the day, job after job, I relish the smells. Fresh-cut grass, blooming flowers, the hint of gasoline on Will after he refills the mower. Gracie complains about the bugs, bees especially. Will repeatedly responds, "No work, no ice skating."

Every time he says it, I think of how lucky I was to have no worries about money. I took for granted that I could take private skating lessons, hire choreographers, buy the best skates, and embellish my dresses with crystals.

The temperature has climbed to 80 degrees, but it seems hotter while I work. I'm swimming in sweat. Gracie's flushed face drips with sweat too.

"Drink your water," I keep telling her.

At the final house—old but well kept—Will plans to trim a boxwood hedge, three rhododendrons, six arborvitae trees, and a Japanese maple tree. Gracie complains she's hot and tired, so he gives me the key to his truck and says, "Start it and put on the AC. Stay in there until it's time to rake." While Gracie plays a game on her phone, I concentrate on Will's arm muscles as he manhandles his hedge clippers. He catches me staring.

I bury my head in my phone and search "boxwood designs," giving myself an excuse for looking in his direction should I need one.

When he's almost done with the job, he signals Gracie and me. We run out to rake and bag the clippings.

Our job ends in the backyard, where Will finishes trimming the last arborvitae. I swig my water and notice a gray metal protrusion against the house. "What's that ugly thing over there?" I ask, pointing, walking to it.

"It's a bulkhead," Will says, following me. "It covers a staircase to the cellar."

Next to it, a large weed taunts me. I sit, grip it, and pull hard, like I'm in a tug-of-war with the earth. "The root won't let go. Must be super deep."

"You really need to get over this weed thing," he says. He trims it to grass level with his weed-snipping power tool.

I pull out a less resistant one. "I've always assumed people hire landscapers to do the whole nine yards, not just specific jobs."

"Now you know, Miss Monroe." He stretches out his hand. I grip it, and he pulls me up.

***

WILL PULLS UP to my house at 5:30 p.m. He tries to hand me fifty dollars, but I refuse to take it.

"Put it toward what I owe you," I say.

"I told you we're square," he says. "You owe me nothing."

"And she's giving me more lessons," Gracie says, "so she doesn't need to give you money, Will."

After Gracie's comment, his brows wrinkle into each other.

"I told her I'd give her a few extra lessons and try to find her an affordable coach." As much as I'd prefer to avoid Nathan for the rest of my life, I can't ignore my discovery: he'd coached his brother, a Special Olympian, ten years ago.

"Thank you," Will says. He plants the money back into my palm. "Would you like to work tomorrow?"

"I have an appointment tomorrow. I can't do anything for about a week," I say. No way Mom will let me work in dirt sooner than that after this biopsy thing.

"What kind of appointment lasts a week?" Will asks. "Never mind. None of my business unless you want a steady job."

Gracie pokes her head between us from the back seat. "A week? Do I have to wait that long for another lesson on the ice?"

"Sorry, Gracie. How about after school next Monday? I'll treat you to a snack in the café after your lesson." I glance at Will. "I'll work Monday morning if you let me leave early for her lesson. Sound good?"

"I need help this week, but okay."

I open the door. "Thanks for letting me work today."

Walking to the side door of my house, I'm thinking, *He probably thinks I'm lazy.* After telling him I was looking for a job, I'm already giving him an excuse as to why I can't work. I want so badly to be honest with him, but this is a guy who maintains a business and takes care of his sister—immense responsibilities. The last thing he needs is a coworker, or girl-friend, who drones on about upcoming medical tests and why she needs them.

Will needs skater Madz. Strong, Madz. Who wants to work. Who wants to love as well.

That Madz can't exist in this shell of me. She needs a

healthy body. The only way to do that is for the doctor to weed this neck lump and mass out of me and fix this glitch in my life.

———

IN THE MUDROOM, I take off my shoes and wash my hands. A "light dinner" awaits me on the kitchen table: a tall glass of iced tea and a small bread pocket stuffed with cheese, tomato, and lettuce.

"Wash those hands," Mom says.

"I did." I collapse into my chair.

"You're feeling better?" my father says.

"I'm dead, but I really liked what I was doing." I add mustard to my sandwich and bite into it.

Mom examines my skin. "You forgot to put on sunblock. You're burnt." She waves her finger at me. "Don't let these kids you're hanging out with—"

"Ava," my father says.

"What, Mason? I just want Madz to remember to put on sunblock. I'm glad she had a good time with the two of them. In fact, I like Gracie."

"I figured you would," I said. Crying, lecturing me in my closet, Gracie megaphoned Mom's voice. "How come no one told me about Nathan's brother?"

"I didn't know Nathan had a brother," Mom says, "and I researched Nathan before hiring him."

"I'm surprised he never told you. I thought you guys were close."

"I talked to him mostly about your skating."

"His name was Oliver, and he was a Special Olympian in

figure skating. Nathan coached him to a gold medal, but shortly after, Oliver died."

Everyone at SuperEdge is caught up in the moment, trying to get through their programs and the drama of the week: who's coaching whom, who's making out with whom, who's going to win the qualifying series of competitions, sectional competitions, and national and world championships. Such distractions keep the spotlight off Nathan's personal life, and I sense he likes it that way. Based on his history of blurting out anything on his mind, if Nathan wanted to talk about Oliver, he would have. He certainly didn't hold back on his "soft and unsuccessful," aka "fat failure," speech to me.

"How did you find out about his brother?" Mom says.

"When I searched for a Special Olympics coach in figure skating for Gracie, Nathan's name popped up. In his brother's obituary." I pull up the website and show her.

A single breath sends another fleeting ache through my chest. Either the obituary is breaking my heart or the mass-thing is saying hello. I eat my little sandwich, drink my iced tea, then head upstairs to shower.

"Don't forget. Nothing to eat or drink after midnight." Mom scoots her chair closer to my father's, and he wraps his arm around her. I love that they like each other.

Will texts: *Since you have the rest of the week off, can I take you out for a little while tonight? I need to tell you something.*

ELEVEN

Other than my make-out sessions with Joao, I've never been in a romantic relationship with a boy, not so much as a date. I've had crushes on a few of my male rink buddies. One was too old for me, another was already dating someone, and another also had a crush on a male rink buddy. Although I'm trying to keep my hopes in check, butterflies are fluttering in my stomach. Maybe he flipped back to wanting to date me, like before our deal.

Starting next week, I'll have the time and mindset to focus on a relationship with him. I already have the feelings: My heart beats faster when I see him. All of my blood rushes to my head when I'm near him. I want to kiss him. I smile when I think of how he cares about others. He went out of his way to bring me a rose after my test, and how sweet is he to help and mentor his sister?

I text Mom: *I'm going out for a little while with Will. If I* had told her any sooner, the odds of my going out would have dropped to nil.

Mom: *??? I'm still upset over what he did.*

Me: :/ *He did it to help me. He wants to talk. I think it's about working with him.*

Mom: *It's 8 o'clock:/ You need to rest. Biopsy tomorrow.*

Me: *Just an hour. He's already here. I can't tell him to leave.* Pressure tactic, applied. Let's see if it works.

Mom: *An hour. That's it.*

I text Will about the time restriction.

He texts back: *Even Cinderella got more time. I'm out front.*

I look out the window at his truck. Frankly, I'm surprised he isn't running in the other direction. On top of everything else that's happened, we're limited to a measly hour. I'd text him my comeback, *Cinderella didn't need to rest for a biopsy,* but why give him another reason to run?

WILL'S pickup truck has been washed inside and out. He earns extra points for replacing the tang of sweat and gasoline with citrusy zest. As I buckle up, I trace the origins of the nose candy to an air freshener clipped to a vent.

"Can I buy you an ice cream?" he asks.

Light supper, nothing after midnight. A cup of soft serve should be okay. "Sure." I look in the back seat, which is empty. "Who's watching Gracie?"

"She's with my mother."

"Does your father live with you?"

"Yeah."

He doesn't offer more information, so I resist asking for it.

Besides, if I ask him a nosey question, he might ask me if the time limit has to do with my "week-long appointment." I look out the window, unable to escape the awkward silence but thrilled to be alone with him in his truck. He supposedly wants to talk to me, yet he doesn't say another word. Until we get to UdderBuds Ice Creamery.

"My treat," he says. "Go crazy."

"I'll have a kiddie-size vanilla soft serve, please."

"I said go crazy, not insane," he whispers. I like the warm tickle of his breath on my cheek. And his voice, so soft and close? Ear candy, compared to his all-business work voice.

"Watch out. I've been known to mix it up and get jimmies," I say. *Ugh.* Aren't I funny?

Once we get our ice cream, we sit in the truck to avoid yellow jackets hunting for a lick. A wad of ice cream tumbles off my spoon, onto my lap. He hands me a napkin. To distract him from my "udder" embarrassment, I say, "You said you wanted to talk to me?"

He pokes his ice cream gently with his plastic spoon until he compiles the perfect mix of nuts, marshmallow, and chocolate ice cream. He holds the spoon in front of my mouth. "Take a walk on the wild side." He pulls the spoon back. "You're not allergic to nuts, are you?"

Here's this guy with a tough edge—intense eyes, muscles, won't budge on the topic of weeds. I don't think he'd put up with crap from anyone. Yet in the dim light, his thick lashes and big brown eyes look especially innocent and doll-like. Every time he blinks, they morph into butterflies. Beautiful black monarchs. I tighten my lips to cork the giggles.

"Not allergic, but I'm good." I giggle. *Rocky Road.* A meltin-your-mouth metaphor. More giggles erupt from mini-earthquakes in my diaphragm. *Stop*, I command myself.

"Glad I'm so entertaining." The spoonful of Rocky Road disappears into his mouth.

The giggling is a nervous tick. It used to torment me right before Joao and I would kiss at the make-out tree.

"It's not you, Will. I'm just"—*don't say it*—"enjoying the poetic simplicity of vanilla bean." There's another giggle. I gave up skating to become the world's worst comedian. I hide my eyes from him, staring at my ice cream as I swirl it around with my spoon.

"I want to talk to you about Gracie," Will says, reviving the dead air. "About your promise to give her extra lessons and find her a coach."

I peek up at him. "Okay."

He wipes his mouth and rests his cup on the dashboard. "I'm sure you meant well. And I don't mean to sound ungrateful. But Gracie remembers things. So if you said what you did to make yourself feel better—"

"What?" I sit up in my seat, squinting.

He holds up his palms. "I mean, to make *her* feel better. If you said it because you thought it would keep her calm or—"

"I meant it."

He sighs, rests his hands on his lap, and gazes out his window. "I don't *expect* people to help her with her skating. My concern is too many people have let Gracie down by breaking promises. Coaches have promised to put her on their waiting list. Gracie would get so excited. Months would go by, then a year, and guess what? We'd watch them take on new students but never Gracie. She notices these things. She's not stupid."

"Do you think her screaming scared them off?"

"Could be, but I think they backed off because she'll never be a star skater like you. High-level skaters are living advertisements for their coaches. Gracie's screaming?" He shakes his head. "Nah. I think the coaches' egos ran interference. Her first coach was decent, but she retired after a few years. A couple of other coaches squeezed her out after a few months by drastically upping their rates."

"I didn't promise her I'd be her forever coach. I was honest about wanting a break from the ice. I already found someone who might—I emphasize *might*—find Gracie a coach with experience teaching Special Olympians figure skating."

"With a committed coach, Gracie can compete outside the Special Olympics. As far as your promises to her, she'll hold you to the plans you made for next Monday but will cut you slack on future lessons. She'd be just as happy if you showed up for a few minutes, once in a while, to watch her, maybe give her a pointer before leaving. Just enough time to let her know you're honoring your promise, that you didn't forget her like others have. For better or worse, you've made an impression on her. She'd be hurt if you fell off the map."

A new kind of pressure adds weight to my mental barbell, and it's the most stressful kind of pressure there is: people counting on me for a moral purpose. I prefer my old skating pressures. At least those can be solved with a clean landing or a bag of ice.

Only I could begin my skating retirement by getting more involved with the skating world.

He shows me the time glowing on his phone. "Ten minutes before my truck turns into a pumpkin and you lose your glass slipper." He reaches his hand out. For a split second, I think he wants to hold mine, but then he says, "Do you want me to toss that?" and takes my trash.

"Thank you."

I watch him walk to the barrel. Then I watch a group of girls watching him walk to the barrel and back to the car. An inkling of pride bubbles up in me for being the one sitting in his truck. At the same time, a slight annoyance festers within me. He, if only for a moment, thought I had reassured Gracie to make myself feel better.

I can't blame him for worrying about his sister's interests, but hasn't he, for one moment, considered my position? I can't be done with skating until I get Gracie a coach and give her a few more lessons. Three, to be exact, because Gracie takes things literally.

I'm locked into a commitment. The thought intimidates me as he drives me home. I offered to help Gracie out of a sense of obligation. She wants to skate; I know how to skate. She wants to compete; I know what it takes to compete. It wouldn't be right if I didn't try to help her.

I guess Will's slip of the tongue revealed the truth. Telling Gracie I'd help her did make me feel better, at least for that moment.

"You're in deep thought. Did I offend you?"

I open my mouth to speak, but he interrupts.

"I can't help it if I'm defensive over my sister. Someone has to watch out for her interests." He pulls into my driveway, hops out, runs to my door, and opens it. Mom's silhouette disappears from the picture window as he walks me to the front door. I keep my head down, feeling guilty over my sense of obligation rather than excitement to help Gracie. She deserves a coach who's excited to get on the ice and train her.

"You didn't offend me," I say. "Not after I thought about it, anyway. I understand you're concerned for your sister."

His fingers gently lift my chin.

Will he or won't he? I'm sure my bout with "the kissing disease" built up a tolerance for it. Does that make me a carrier? His gaze wanders from my eyes to my lips.

"Good night," he says. His eyes return to mine, and he steps back.

No need to worry about kissing diseases tonight. I reach for the door handle, hanging on to it as I watch him.

Chin down, hands in his pockets, he skips down the stairs, kicks a stone down the walkway, and gets into his truck. When its rattling fades away, the fluttering in my stomach turns to churning as the butterflies of love flutter down a deep, dark hole known as the Friend Zone.

I'm not likable.

I may not be Miss USA, and I may have a nervous laugh, but I think I have more to offer than that mean girl who wore high heels to the rink. I go inside the house.

"Why do you look so down?" Mom asks.

Because my sort-of-relationship is fizzling out. "Who's down?" I kiss her good night.

The fizzling out's probably a good thing. Why put myself through another boyfriend lecture? My parents are still recovering from the Joao saga, which landed me a lot of swollen glands, throat cultures, and for all I know, tomorrow's biopsy. I peek into my father's office. His desk lamp spotlights his face with a soft glow.

"Why are you in here so late?" I ask him.

His eyes hurdle his readers. "Getting my morning work done. I'm going with you and your mother tomorrow."

"Wow, you're really stepping out of the zone. Two family outings within a few days of each other." I blow him a kiss. "I'm glad you'll be there, Dad."

He blows me a kiss.

Mom walks me to my room. "Are you scared about tomorrow?"

A good way to scare a person is to ask, *Are you scared?* "Should I be?"

She bites her bottom lip.

Now there's a pep talk. I can't tell if she's being her usual overly nervous self or if this is appropriate nervousness I should be feeling too. "The procedure tomorrow is a minor one, right?"

She sews her eyebrows so tight she may need a seam ripper to separate them. She smiles, hugs me, kisses my head, and hugs me again.

"Mom, you're scaring me with all this . . . warmth."

"I just want you to know I love you. And you're right. This is a minor procedure. People get biopsies all the time." She kisses my cheek. "Good night, baby." That should do it, but she hangs on.

"Mom."

"Okay, good night. I love you."

TWELVE

I awaken to a mixture of monitor beeping and people mumbling, but my eyes insist upon playing dead.

"Madzy," Mom's voice says.

My lids flicker open to a massive blur, and I'm pretty sure I'm dreaming. Hearing beeping, I squint, looking for the source. Pink-and-blue hues come into view. A set of eyes meet mine in a gap between the wall and the striped curtain. She's another patient, lying on a stretcher. Someone pulls the curtain to the wall, breaking our connection.

I close my eyes again. A tear drips down my cheek, and I sniffle. More tears pool and drip onto my pillowcase. I have no idea why I'm crying.

"It's okay," Mom says, dabbing my cheeks with what must be a tissue but scratches like a napkin-notebook-paper hybrid. I drift off, lulled by monitor-beeping, a warm blanket . . . darkness . . .

"Deep breaths, Madelyn," a male voice says. I inhale

deeply through my mouth, bypassing my stuffy nose. "We're boosting you up in the stretcher. Can you turn on your back?"

Uh, no, I'm sleeping. Oh, I get it. The procedure's over.

"C'mon, Madz. Deep breath again. Bend those legs and push up on three. One, two . . ."

Really, people? What kind of medical professionals anesthetize you and then immediately put you to work? Last I heard, operating under the influence was a bad thing. I reach for my nose to scratch an itch, but my finger hits an oxygen mask and my IV tubing tugs on the back of my hand. I follow the tubing, which disappears under the covers. I try to turn onto my side and free the tubing from the weight of my covers, but wires sprouting from my chest snag me. I'm entwined in the clutches of a giant squid.

"Let's take this off." Male Voice pulls the mask off my face, and I open my eyes. My parents are wrinkled-brow bookends at the foot of the bed. The guy nurse covers me with a heated blanket and shows me the call bell at the tip of a tentacle twisted around the bed rail.

My parents move in unison to my side. Dad's hairy knuckles hook around the rail. My eyes hike up his wedding ring, then up his tall, heavyset frame to his face, which always makes me feel at home even when I'm not. His eyes grab hold of mine, and he offers me a sturdy nod that relays, *Yup, we're F-ed, but the force about to take us down can't contend with the fortitude behind this nod.* He sweeps my hair away from my face like he did when I was little and he tucked me in.

"We have good news and bad news," he says. "The bad news is you have cancer. Hodgkin's lymphoma. The biopsy results were called into the OR while you were still under anesthesia. The good news is it's curable." He smiles. "And that's not just good news; it's great news." He kisses my forehead.

If it's great news, why is Mom crying? They aren't tears of joy. The corners of her mouth are drooping.

My mind struggles to catch up with the awake world, where there seems to be some sort of mix-up. "My neck lump was cancer?"

"Yes," Dad says.

"But the doctor removed it. So I'm good, right?"

Dad strokes my head as if I'm a wounded puppy. "You have other suspicious lymph nodes in your neck."

"And in your chest," Mom says. She wraps her fingers around my fingers, the ones on the hand with the IV.

"Lymph nodes in my chest?"

"Yes," Dad says. "Remember the good news. It *is* curable."

Mom's smile is a facial twitch. It's an improvement from the first time Dad mentioned the good news. Nevertheless, her inability to drum up a real smile reminds me there's a hitch.

Dad sits in a chair next to the stretcher. "You'll need chemotherapy, and depending on how you respond to it, you may or may not need a small dose of radiation for insurance."

The surgeon shows up and tells me we were lucky I got the neck-lump biopsy results so quickly. It allowed him to biopsy my bone marrow and insert a portacath while I was still under anesthesia. He claims my veins are small, and the port will make administering my treatments easier. "The site may be sore for a few days."

"More aches," I mumble.

"You'll get over this, Madz," the surgeon says. "This is one of the better cancers to get." He offers Mom the same cliché nod my father gave me.

Better cancers? How is one better than the other? They all eat away at your body until they freaking kill you. That's what Lindsey told me, anyway, when her grandmother died from it. I didn't fact-check her. At the time, the subject didn't affect me.

Groggy from the anesthetic lingering in my system, I close my eyes, tempted to fall back asleep. I open my eyes to Mom. She presses a tissue against her nose, her eyes running water like spigots. *This isn't real,* I tell myself, sure I'm dreaming. *This isn't real.*

THE ATMOSPHERE WEIGHS heavy in front of the pediatric hospital, whose sidewalk is a pedestrian freeway more dizzying than the congested street. Everyone whips past me as I sit in a haze of car exhaust and human breath. One way or another, we're all in a fog. I am, Mom is, and passersby, absorbed in their own problems, are.

I weep, unable to stop the slow, steady leak. The surgeon told me anesthesia affects some people like this, but I have other reasons to cry. On the upper right side of my chest, my fingers rest on a bump. It's the portacath the surgeon implanted for my impending chemo treatments. "Why me?" slips out of my mouth.

"That's what I keep thinking. Why you? Why couldn't it be *me?*" Mom buries her face in tissue again.

The thought of her getting sick switches my thinking. *Thank God it's me.* I couldn't handle losing my parents. I wipe my eyes with a remnant of tissue. Dad says my problem is curable. If true, then I have to believe I can get through this. I'll have to convey that to my parents so they don't worry themselves to death.

Dad pulls up to the curb. The patient care assistant wheels me to the car and helps me in. Mom sits in the back seat with me, a rare thing because she gets car sick back here. She slips a motion-sickness pill into her mouth.

I'm disconnected from myself, here and not here at the same time. Like this person sitting next to her mother and behind her father isn't me. "Slide over a little more, Madz . . . Buckle up . . . Let me help you." Mom tells me what to do, and I do it. I'm a puppet going through the motions.

What's worse, I'm the cause of her tears. Whether she's expressing sympathy or fear, I'd rather she keep a stiff upper lip and tell me to "suck it up" as she did at the rink, her way of toughening me up. The funny thing is she'd crinkle her brow and glue her eyes to me for the rest of the session as if she couldn't take her own advice.

I doze in the car, so we're home in a blink. Dad drops Mom and me off at the front of the house. "I'll be back in an hour," he says, taking off to check a construction site.

The walk to the front door re-orients my feet to gravity, and I no longer feel as though I'll float away like a balloon loosed to the wind. As I step inside the house, someone in the entryway mirror captures my attention. She stares at me. I inch closer to her, focusing on a pencil-thin line low on her neck.

I place my fingers on the clear film covering the incision above my collarbone. "No more bump."

"Don't touch it," Mom says.

My eyes return to the girl in the mirror, the one who, if I look close enough, resembles me. A bony, sallow, scary-old-doll version of me. "Where did I go?" I whisper.

In the living room, Gallagher lays my pillow and cotton quilt on the couch.

"I'd rather rest on the couch in the gazebo," I say.

"Whatever you want, love," he says.

"I'll take them," Mom says, grabbing the pillow and quilt.

We walk outside to the screened-in gazebo, where I won't have to wrestle with bugs.

A few minutes later, Gallagher comes in and sets down a tray with a bottle of water, a cup of yogurt with fresh fruit, a cup of tea, and a piece of pound cake.

"Thanks, Gallagher," I say as he leaves.

"It's cool in here with the fan going." Mom unfurls the quilt and covers my legs.

"Don't tell anyone except Gallagher what the doctor said," I tell her. "I don't want people forecasting my death before I even start my first treatment."

She sits next to me. "Can I tell Lindsey's mother? She texted me, asking how your biopsy turned out."

"I guess, but tell her after my scan and wait till I'm cured before you tell anyone else." A PET-CT at Haven Shore Cancer Institute will map out and stage the cancer. I'm hoping it's perfect and proves my biopsy was a false positive. The scan is scheduled for tomorrow.

"What if my sister or your father's brother calls and asks for you?"

Her sister lives in New Zealand, and my uncle on my father's side is a confirmed bachelor traveling the world. "Okay, but no one else. I'm serious."

She runs her hand over my head, calming me. "Whatever you want."

"It's what I need." I'm still not 100 percent convinced I've been diagnosed correctly. Three strikes, and I'll buy the diagnosis of Hodgkin's lymphoma. Strike one is the chest X-ray showing a mass in my chest; strike two, the biopsy; strike three, Thursday's PET-CT.

Pulling up my quilt, I turn on my side and drift off to sleep.

RAINDROPS PATTER AGAINST THE GAZEBO, real rain that, unlike the top ranker on my soothing-sounds playlist, offers a corresponding soothing smell. I breathe in, savoring the misty mixture of water and earth served on a gentle breeze. No better way to wake up. I pull my quilt higher up, covering half my face. Gallagher comes in, hands Mom an umbrella, and grabs my tray.

"Let's go, kiddo," Mom says.

"Can I sleep out here tonight? I'll need another blanket."

"No way. A thunderstorm is brewing. Let's go in before it starts."

I sit up slowly. The incisions pull, and I wince.

"Are you in pain?" Mom asks.

"I'm okay." Sore with every move, I wrap the quilt around my shoulders and follow her out of the gazebo.

She opens the umbrella, wraps an arm around me, and the three of us hurry to the house.

Mom shakes out the umbrella while I open the fridge and stare. "What am I looking for?"

"Not sure," she says, shutting the French doors, "but I know what Gracie's looking for. You. While you slept, she lit up your phone with messages." She hands me my cell.

And then there's that. Commitments don't disappear just

because I have . . . I don't want my commitment to disappear. I refuse to let whatever's wrong with me interfere with my life. I made a promise to Will, dammit. It's one thing to hold back information, like my illness; it's another to go back on my word. He'll hate me. He'll think I'm a phony and a liar, yet another coach who hurt Gracie by failing to keep a promise.

Frig cancer.

Text after text, Gracie asks if I can teach her Friday, as I did last week.

I can't go on the ice with fresh incisions. I'd teach from the boards if it didn't require fielding questions about why I'm not on the ice. Sitting at the table, cocooned in my quilt, I text her: *I told you I can't teach you until Monday. Remember? I'm really busy this week. Sorry if you misunderstood.*

Thursday, after my PET-CT, I'll meet my oncologist at Haven Shore's pediatric clinic. With those things hanging over my head, it's hard to concentrate on concocting excuses that will answer Gracie's questions without hurting her.

Gracie texts me again: *What r u doing? Why r u busy? Did u go back to skating?*

Me: *Didn't go back to skating, and sorry, can't text. My mother's calling me.* My equivocating has officially turned into lying.

Lying is a toxic condition in its own right. If tomorrow's scan backs up my cancer diagnosis, I'll have to figure out how to tell Gracie the truth without giving away too much of the truth. Until this nightmare is behind me. For now, the less I text her, the better.

There's no easy way out of this, but there's no way I'll let people see me as a dead person walking. I know what people think when they hear the C-word. They think what I thought and what Lindsey will think if her mother tells her. *When* her mother tells her, I should say.

Lindsey texts me a heart.

Mom ratted me out. I knew she wouldn't wait until after the PET-CT.

I text Lindsey: *I'm sure your mother told you, so don't tell me she didn't.*

Lindsey: *She did.*

Me: *You can't tell anyone. Please. And what happened to your grandmother won't happen to me, so don't worry. I'll get through this.*

Lindsey: *I won't tell anyone.*

She's never texted so little. By not commenting on my comment about getting through this, she gives the impression she doesn't think I will. She could be unsure of what to say. If I were her, I might be at a loss for words too. I would offer some form of moral support, such as, "Of course you'll get through this, Madz; you're a fighter." Then again, I left SuperEdge after a fall that caused a mere bruise. Why would she think I'm a fighter?

My father isn't a liar. He wouldn't say my supposed cancer is curable if it weren't. Its curability makes Hodgkin's a "better cancer," according to the doctor. This "good news" leads me to believe I can simultaneously fight this beast growing inside me and keep my commitment to Will and Gracie.

"Take a break, Gallagher," Mom says. She hands him a cup of tea before bringing hers to the table.

I look up from my phone. "You told Lindsey's mother already, but I forgive you because I know you're having a rough day. Because of me."

"I wouldn't exactly put it that way, but thank you." She sits next to me. "Can I tell Nathan?"

"Of course not. Why, of all people, would you want to tell him?" Bad enough I have to text him. I've put it off but can't much longer.

"Please stop cracking your knuckles." She rests her hands on mine. "Nathan has been an active part of our lives for six years. He should know why you've been so tired. That you haven't been making it up."

He's been active in our lives because she paid him. *Don't go there,* I tell myself. I won't expend energy on a dead-end conversation bound to hurt her feelings. "Think about what you're saying, Mom. Did I need to get cancer to legitimize my fatigue?" I close my eyes in a lame attempt to swat the sting of tears. "I was training six days a week."

She sighs, says, "I'm sorry," and follows me upstairs.

I could use my diagnosis to deliver a whopping "I told you so" to Nathan and guilt him into helping me: *Turns out my "laziness" was cancer, Nathan. I could really use your help while I'm battling for my life. Would you find a proper coach for my friend?*

No way. I'd be seeking exactly what I'm intent on dodging: pity and projections of death. If enough people think I'm a goner, it could happen.

"I'll never forgive you if you tell him," I say to Mom. "If I really do have cancer, I'm going to kick its ass. Then I'll finish my last few high school classes and apply to colleges. I can't accomplish those things knowing everyone's gossiping about whether or not I'm going to die."

"Stop saying things like that." She dabs her eyes.

"Is everything okay up there?" Dad calls up the stairs.

"Everything's great, Dad."

When I text Nathan for help with Gracie, he won't know I have cancer but should respond right away regardless. If he didn't block me. He's been in the trenches I'm in now. He had to navigate a path to success in figure skating for someone he cared about. He understood his brother deserved a chance at success like everyone else.

"We'll tell him about my cancer after I'm cured or close to it," I say to Mom. I open a window, lean on the sill, and focus on the living: two birds bathing in a puddle by the pool, rain lightly showering them. It's also watering the stupid dandelions popping up around the poolhouse. Again.

Mom stands beside me and looks out the window. I lean my head on her shoulder. "You did a good job designing the backyard," she says. "I think of you when I look at it. I remember why you placed everything where you did."

"I loved planning it." Designing a yard is like painting a picture I can literally bring to life. I straighten out, determined to plan for my future. "I'm going to research colleges, then take a nap. I'll see you at supper."

Rivers of grief run down her cheeks.

"Don't cry." Here's a terrible admission: her weeping annoys me. "If you cry, I'm gonna think you're expecting me to die." I hug her. "I need you solid. No tears. Good vibes."

In spite of my stinging eyes, I firmly hold back my own tears. The Hoover Dam has nothing on Madz Monroe.

PART 2
"BRUISES"

THIRTEEN

Propped up on pillows and stretched across my bed Wednesday morning, I search for colleges offering degrees in landscape architecture. Thunder rumbles as I open a window to colleges with the best programs. A southern college would be a more practical option than a school in New England. In the south, snow is less likely to interfere with landscaping projects. My favorite on this particular list is a college in Georgia. I savor the lick of hope it gives me and move on.

I research *spiral*—the kind skaters perform, not the metaphorical downward kind I'm caught up in. When Gracie asked me why it's named that, I gave her Nathan's demonstrable answer: regardless of body position, if I hold an edge long enough, it will curve inward and carve a spiral pattern in the ice. My search proves that answer correct but doesn't explain why the spiral move is named a spiral.

The sky cracks and booms, kicking off the search *Why is a spiral named a spiral in figure skating?* I pull the covers over my head and skim the top results. In summary, spirals are named according to the direction the skater's gliding in, the edge she's moving on, and the free-leg position, which is always above the hip. I entered the search with the arabesque spiral in mind, the one similar to the ballet move. The skater glides on one edge across the ice, body horizontal to the ice, chin up, arms out, free leg raised behind like she's pretending to fly. The body lines are smooth and graceful, as the name, arabesque, implies.

Searching for spiral images, I find dizzying designs drawn by people, and swirling, sparkling patterns drawn by the heavens. Some spirals lie flat, some spiral down, and some spiral up. Those on a flat plane remind me of the swirl my blade carves on the ice when I enter a spin.

Bingo. There's another lesson for Gracie—the spiral motion of the edge, how it drives us into a spin, and how we can study the marking on the ice to check if a spin is centered. I'll show her after I heal. I'll also answer her question better about the naming of spirals relative to body position.

Autism. I've heard the expression "Autism speaks." Based on my experience with Gracie, I'd assert autism yells. Another tidbit of information leads me to think, *Don't assert or assume anything.* Autism is really *Autism Spectrum Disorder,* "spectrum" indicating symptoms range from mild to severe; care level, one to three. Gracie must be mild, level one on the spectrum. Other than her difficulty lacing and her disregard for rink etiquette, she seems pretty normal.

Normal. I suppose that runs on a spectrum too.

I may have to call Will. He told me not to give Gracie too much information at once or she'll get frustrated. "Her auditory processing trips up," he said. Easy enough, but how tough of a coach should I be? How hard should I push her? I wouldn't want to destroy Gracie's love of skating by being too tough or stunt her progress by not being tough enough. I'd feel that way about any student I were to teach.

Hodgkin's lymphoma . . . my head can only absorb so much in one morning.

I wash down two acetaminophens with water and sit on my chaise longue, pronounced "shaze lon" à la française, how we classy rich people say it. Especially when we're bored.

My parents told me to rest until tomorrow, the day we return to the hospital for my PET-CT and doctor appointment. How do I rest with a sore chest (thanks to my newly placed port) and more tests and appointments hanging over my head? A friendly distraction would improve the situation, but such a distraction is a thing of the past.

My phone's a bee that lost its buzz.

Am I not worthy of even one *What's up?* I set it to ping last night at seven to prevent myself from constantly checking for messages. Sixteen hours later, pingless. My intuition was spot on. The people I've skated with at SuperEdge aren't my friends. They're coworkers. Peers. Rink mates. But not *friends*.

Before I broke loose from SuperEdge, their texts were like daily journal entries—rink gossip, progress reports on their skating, pictures of new skating dresses, plans for coordinating our practice attire, upcoming competitions, test results. What do we have in common outside the rink? Would they be interested in my incisions or my treatment plan?

I expected more from Lindsey, who has gone AWOL. No doubt she's skating, rebounding from her injury, trying to impress Nathan—back to usual. The difference? Her usual used to include texting me morning, noon, and night. Is she avoiding me, unsure of what to say because she thinks I'll suffer the same fate as her grandmother? Could she have flipped like the others, fearful Nathan would shun her for associating with me?

I text Lindsey: *Hi [happy face emoji]. I hope your back is feeling good and your skating is going well:)*

I text Gracie: *Hi [waving-hand emoji]* to let her know I haven't forgotten her. She should be home from school by now.

I set my phone on the marble table beside me, sitting in a position I've yet to find comfortable: unsure of what to do next. Wincing, I reach for the book Gallagher gave me for my birthday six months ago, *Forever Emerald: Landscapes of Ireland.* The binding cracks as I open it. I've been meaning to read it but never had the time. Mom calls it a coffee-table book. Makes sense. It's too large to fit comfortably on a bookshelf. I slide my fingertips over a cool, smooth page.

The heavy paper makes flipping through the book a breeze, but I take my time scanning each page. A two-page spread shows sheep, round and puffy like cotton balls, dotting lush-green hills. No weeds, of course—the sheep gobble them up. In the background, a stone castle crumbles on its emerald bed, a shell of what it used to be on the majestic hill. Another page holds a gray sky whose tones saturate the seascape below it. A cliff holds back the massive tide. The full-color picture may as well be black and white. I don't see what's so "emerald" about that, but this is only one picture, and if you look hard enough, you can imagine the emerald in the ocean.

After flipping through all the pages, I flip back to the beginning of the book and read the text describing the pictures, lulling myself into another nap.

FOURTEEN

Sunlight leaks through cracks in the curtains, gold-washing the soft curves of my silky pink drapes and adding a twinkle to the mini chandelier in the center of my room. The sky cried every tear it had. Now, the sun beams down an invitation to get outside and live.

My brain tells me to go outside, but instead, I pick on lunch. As with breakfast, Gallagher brought it to my room. I take a bite out of my hummus wrap, finish a banana, and shortly after, my body sinks into sleep again. I follow this dozing-waking pattern throughout the rest of the afternoon, which passes by in a slow-motion time-lapse.

As the sun arcs closer to the horizon, a body of shade moves like a giant monster. It slugs up the wall and across the ceiling, where it eventually slurps up the shimmer of crystals dangling from my chandelier.

The shadow engulfing me rattles me, reminding me it's 7 p.m. and I'm wasting time. I pick my coffee-table book off the floor, return it to the table, and take my phone. It springs to life with a ping.

Lindsey: *Back is good, and the ice is awesome! (New doors in rink) I landed all of my singles with no pain. [muscle emoji] Will work on doubles tomorrow finally. Hope that chest-mass thing isn't bothering you too much:)*

I switch the notification ping back to vibrate now that I know the phone's working. Another text arrives: *Hey, it's Will. Gracie can't text. She's doing homework.*

Me: *You sound like you're her father lol.*

Him: *May as well be. I'll have her text you in an hour. Can I call you?*

May as well be her father? My thumbs twitch, itching to hop on that Pandora's box of a comment. Uh-uh, won't even jiggle the lock. We barely register on the friendometer. I text him back *Sure.*

Seconds later, my phone buzzes. "Hi," I say.

"Hey."

"Aren't you bothering Gracie by talking?"

"I went outside. How's your week-long appointment going? Off to a good start?"

"Just dandy." *Ugh*, I actually said that. "Can you do me a favor? It doesn't involve money. I promise." A glimpse across the room at my bureau mirror turns into a stare.

. . .

"Waiting," he says.

"Make sure Gracie does her off-ice exercises. She'll know what I'm talking about." I study my reflection, continuing my search for an inkling of me.

"I know what you're talking about too. I've overheard

enough skating moms to know about off-ice training, test levels, all that stuff."

"Good. Text me her summer skating schedule. Tell her I'll text her at the end of the week." My heart gallops like a wild horse as I consider slipping down May As Well Be Lane. After all, we're talking, he's sharing, and I fear his may-as-well-be comment was a cry for help. In a normal situation, a seventeen-year-old boy doesn't parent his sister.

"I'll text it to you now. Talk to you later."

Wait. The word rides up my throat but screeches to a stop at my lips. I bite them. *Self-control, Madz.* I'm walking that fine line between showing I care and coming across as nosey.

"Okay. Bye." I suck in a deep breath—ouch—and exhale like I'm blowing out birthday candles. My pounding heart slows to steady thumps. Talking to Will gets my blood pumping. Initially, I blamed the nerves of a crush. Lately, I blame the nerves of fear.

I'm afraid of letting him down by failing his sister and breaking his trust in me. Another part of me worries he'll let me down. If I tell him the truth about my situation, he might pity me. And I might hate him for it.

I rest my phone on its charger and gravitate to my full-length mirror, hoping to find a better reflection. Some mirrors are more flattering than others—it's a thing. Usually, this mirror works with the natural light streaming in, highlighting my eyes with a twinkle and my cheeks and lips with pink hues. But now, a grayish hue contours my face, my eyes sink into dark pits, and my pale skin pops from the shadows.

I'm skin and bones. Nathan was right. I did lose too much weight. The ghost of me grows as I float closer to the mirror. Closer to the incision over my collarbone, covered by a clear film. I pull my V-neck to the side, exposing another incision below the collarbone, near the portacath bump.

My fingertips slide over swollen lymph nodes along the sides of my throat. Damn. They're like strands of pearls, sandwiching my throat, except for one lump on the right side. It's more like a budding golf ball. I swear these things popped up overnight.

The timing of my UdderBuds tête-à-tête with Will was good. Better we did it pre-biopsy. My current appearance would push the limits of a running theme: he always sees me at my worst. I sit on my bed.

"Eat your supper, love," Gallagher says, peeking into my room. He comes in holding a tray with a small dish of carrot sticks and a dish covered with a silver dome. "It's seven o'clock. You're running late, sleepy head. C'mon." He puts the tray on my bedside table.

I don't dare lift the dome in front of him. The odor coming from it will explode in my face, and I'll gag. "You're running late too. You didn't stay on duty just to bring me this, did you?"

"That I did, love. You can thank me by eating it all up. I'm going home now. Goodnight, my dear."

Gallagher's home is within my home. His apartment is off the kitchen. I like having him around, and that Irish brogue of his? Everything he says sounds pleasant. If he were to swear, even that would sound sweet: "Freak you, love. You're quite the arsehole, my dear." The house would feel empty without him.

On the other side of the bed, I open the window by the table my phone is charging on. The mirror warned me I might have more of a battle on my hands than I thought. As a result, my need to text Nathan has grown more urgent. I reach for the phone as if I'm about to touch metal after rubbing my feet on a rug. *Gracie deserves a proper coach,* I tell myself. *Who's experienced in teaching kids with neurodevelopmental issues.*

I need that coach as well. ASAP. A consistent coach for Gracie would distract her and Will from my absence and broken promises. This would lighten the impact on Gracie's psyche—she won't miss the lessons I promised her. Will might be less forgiving. All he wants me to do is keep my Monday promise to Gracie and, after that, watch her skate once in a while so she won't think I forgot her. I plan to watch her when I'm better. Until then, her having a suitable, consistent coach will lighten the burden on Will even if he's upset with me.

Facing the open window, I sit on the floor. My reluctant thumbs manage to construct a sincere and professional text. After a half hour and several drafts, I text Nathan the following:

Hi, I hope you're well. I'm wondering if you know anyone who could coach a friend of mine. Her name is Gracie. She's fourteen, has challenges on the autism spectrum, takes direction well, and is eager to learn. She loves skating, wants to compete, and passed her pre-tests. I noticed you coached your late (so sorry for your loss) brother through the Special Olympics in figure skating, which is why I'm asking you. I know you have a busy schedule, but I'm hoping you can squeeze in a reply. Thanks in advance for your help.

I tap *send,* unsure if the message will get to him. If he didn't block me, either a cosmic shift occurred or my hypothesis was correct: he wouldn't block me out of respect for Mom.

"Madz."

I jerk my head in Mom's direction, the twisting skin sending zings through my incisions. "Ow."

"Sorry, honey. Didn't mean to scare you."

"Scare me? I'm lucky my incisions didn't split open." I peek down my shirt to make sure the portacath's okay. It is. I walk to my mirror and check my neck incision. No blood, edges still stuck together, puffy. I run my finger along it.

"Ooh, don't touch it," Mom says. "Does it feel okay?"

"Weird, but okay."

"That's good because I'd like you to bring what's left of your supper downstairs. Dad and I are eating late, too, and want you to sit with us." Normally, she's in Dad's office at this time, complaining about a client and sipping on her Pinot Grigio.

"I'm fine up here. Gallagher set me up. I'll watch TV with you later on."

She wraps her arms around me, kisses my cheek, and we look at each other in the mirror. "Please come sit with us. We miss you. We wove our wittle Madzy." She presses her lips against my cheek and plants ten tiny kisses on it. I understand her urge to nurture, but she's doing it with the fervor of Norman Bates's mother. If this is going to be an ongoing thing while I'm sick, I'll have to set some ground rules.

I give in to her request. However, her jack-in-the-box dinner announcement aggravated my incisions. Due for my pain medicine, I pop a couple of acetaminophens, asking myself if I'll ever again experience comfort or robust health. Mononucleosis, contusions, exhaustion, surgery—I've had enough "bugs" infesting my life lately. It's time for a fumigation.

NATHAN'S TEXT: *So Miss Skating's A Job isn't quite done with figure skating.* Right there. That's why he didn't block me. His jabs are out-of-tune strums on my mental guitar strings, and he's not done messing with my head.

You're doing this for Gracie, I tell myself.

"No phones at the table, Madz," Dad says. "We want to see that beautiful face of yours."

"It's Nathan," I say.

Like sensor-controlled yard lamps, Mom's baby blues light up at the sound of his name.

"He didn't block you." She smiles. "So sweet." She lifts her wineglass to her lips and takes a happy sip.

My parents' eyes meet in a mutual licking of the chops, and I'm not talking about the ones Gallagher steeped in garlic and herbs to mask the death stench. I lay the phone beside my plate and lift the silver dome covering my zucchini quiche, usually my favorite non-vegan meal. It reeks. I think Gallagher got into a batch of bad eggs. I push it away and pick on my dish of carrot sticks.

"And?" Mom says, skewering a piece of pork.

"And what?"

"What did Nathan say?"

"Nothing helpful. I asked him about Gracie, but he gave me attitude." Attitude I consciously removed myself from Friday and will only deal with for Gracie's sake.

Mom and Dad share a glance before their eyes return to their plates. Mom forks another piece of chop and gingerly places it into her mouth, airing faux nonchalance.

My powers weaken as my mind smolders in disgruntlement over Nathan's dig. "You'd think he wouldn't play head games with this one. I mean, Gracie really wants this, and he's taught kids with unique learning styles. If he can't invest the time, I'm sure he knows someone who can."

"Let's just worry about getting you better," Mom says. "I'm sure Nathan will help. He's giving you attitude because he's hurt. He'll come around."

"You know, Mom, I think you care more about his feelings than mine." I lift my hands to my mouth and gag. "Why did Gallagher give me rotten eggs?"

Mom covers the quiche with the silver dome. "Shh. He'll hear you." She points to the open door of his living quarters. "He made that quiche especially for you, and the eggs aren't bad. It's your hyperosmia acting up." She taps the corners of her mouth with her napkin. "I don't care more about Nathan's feelings than yours." She moves to the seat next to me and rubs my back. "Why are you stressing yourself out over this girl? She'll never be able to skate at your level, and you know Nathan trains elite skaters."

"I'm not stressing myself out. Nathan's stressing me out. Of all people, I thought he would understand. His brother—" Elbows on the table, I plant my face in my hands.

"No need to cry over this, Madz," Dad says.

"I'm not crying. I'm moping."

"Well, then, no need to mope," he says. "Nathan will find someone for Gracie if I have to speak to him myself about it. If he doesn't find someone, I will." He leans toward me from his end-of-the-table, king-of-the-house seat and softly cups my chin in his hand. "How's that, sugarplum?"

Yes. I've been dealt the *sugarplum* card, and I'm playing it. "Thank you, Daddy." Although cringeworthy to call him that at my age, *Daddy* is a key component of my sugarplum-card rocking. I hug him, grateful to have an insurance policy in place for

Gracie's training. "Make sure you tell him Gracie doesn't have much money, okay?"

"Okay, sweetie. Now please eat something."

"Okay, Dad." Only one *Daddy* per sugarplum.

I whip my head around, and again the incision stings. "Gallagher," I say. As usual, he left the door to his apartment ajar. He pokes his head out. "Never mind. Sorry." He's off duty, about as much as a grandfather would be. This fills a gap left by both sets of my grandparents, who no longer reside among the living. Although he has his own living quarters, he often eats with us and sometimes watches a movie with us in our home theater. A couple of times, he came on vacation with us.

I scurry to the fridge and check the date on the eggs . . . The sell-by date is ten days away. *Ugh.* Mom's right. My hyperosmia has kicked into full gear. I'm scenting the egg-version smell of death, pre-chick remains. "Sorry, little chickie," I mumble, grabbing a cup of chocolate pudding.

I return to the table, where my face-down phone vibrates with a notification. Mom sits straight up as if startled. I refuse to check the message because I owe my father this pudding cup.

"Is it Nathan? You should answer if it's him." Mom points to the clock. "He's between sessions now. He only has five or ten min—"

"Ava, let it go," Dad says. "It's a text, not a phone call." He winks at me as Mom finishes her last gulp of Pinot and measures another six ounces. She usually restricts herself to no more than five ounces a night, minus Mondays, Tuesdays, and Thursdays, her wine-free days. But it looks like she's going for a Wobbly Wednesday. My father's eyes bob from her wineglass to her. "If you're going to drink that, don't complain about dizziness tonight."

"I'll drink a glass of water before going to bed."

The woman's got a strategy for everything. I'm about to check my message when Gallagher leaves his apartment, sniffling, holding a teacup. He sits at the little table by the pantry and sips his tea. I go to him and softly rest my hand on his back. "Sorry about the drama. Did we make it impossible for you to hear your show?"

"No, love," Gallagher says. "Just thinking about how big you're getting, coming into your own. I'm glad you're making new friends." He nods with a smile, his cheeks extra pink.

I used to think Gallagher blushed a lot, but when I brought it up, he said, "It's the sugar." His nightly beer with dinner doesn't help the situation. I said that to him after finding out he had diabetes. He said, "I cut out enough from my diet. Why live if I can't have a measly beer with my supper?"

I thought, *Jeez, Gallagher, all you have to do is practice a little self-control. Is one beer worth your health?* But now I'm thinking, *Go for it.* Not much is guaranteed in life. If a single beer secures him a few moments of enjoyment each day, why not have one?

"You should walk with me sometime," I say to him. I want him around for a long time. My father too. I turn my head to him, pulling my incision again. "You, too, Dad—"

I gasp and point to Mom. "I saw you looking at that." I stomp to the table and grab my phone.

"Ava, what's wrong with you?" Dad says.

Mom leans on the table, goblet in hand. "I didn't see anything." She sips her vino. "I don't think it's right to bother

Nathan about this. He already has a full schedule and a waiting list to boot."

"One could argue I opened up a spot for Gracie."

She huffs, grabs her briefcase from the doorway, and stomps through the French doors leading to the patio. Her daughter just got a cancer diagnosis, and she's pissed over Gracie taking my place at SuperEdge.

Dad's eyes pop up from his plate. "You don't have to rub salt in the wound. She's very proud of your skating."

I plop into my seat and cross my arms. "Yeah, of my skating."

He points his fork at me. "Of you. Of all the time and hard work you put into the sport, how beautifully you skated, all you've achieved. Give her some time. Deal?"

A heavy sigh ends with my response, "Deal."

Making deals: the adopted inevitability of my life.

FIFTEEN

Thursday morning I'm a human specimen. The PET-CT tech sticks me three times, attempting to start an IV. (The third time it works.) She claims she's new to the job and doesn't want to "play around" with my port without an RN nearby. After the scan, I check in to see Dr. Mu, my oncologist, and find out I must first get a cardiac echo, an ultrasound of my heart.

In a dark room, the technician presses a goo-slathered wand onto my chest and slides it around to "check how the ticker's working." When she's done, she leads me into Dr. Mu's office.

"We're lucky the scheduler fit all these appointments into one day," Mom tells me.

"The faster we do the groundwork," Dad says, "the quicker we can get you healthy again."

They have a point. Every test I get done is a step forward on the path to recovery.

Dr. Mu's medical student goes on a lymph-node fishing

expedition, poking around my neck, pits, belly, and groin, feeling for lumps. Been there, done that. I put up with it because I'm contributing to the future of medicine.

She sits with Dr. Mu before the computer, studying my PET-CT scan, a 3-D map of cancer hotspots. Mine, including the mass in my chest, light up above the diaphragm, consistent with stage IIA Hodgkin's lymphoma. The biopsy validates the scan findings and vice versa. Meaning: I definitely have the big C. Which really pisses me off.

Really, God? I have plans.

"Good news," Dr. Mu says. "Your cancer stage is favorable. Often, weight loss indicates the unfavorable stage, but yours doesn't fit the criteria. You haven't lost at least ten percent of your weight over six months. You lost a few pounds last year from mono and strep throat, then a few more during your last bout of strep throat, in November."

"Strep would make my throat so sore I could hardly swallow."

He nods. "Your skating schedule, combined with the worsening of your hyperosmia, could have triggered your recent weight loss of a few more pounds." Holding his stethoscope, he approaches me.

"She's not training anymore, Doctor," Mom says. "That should help."

Well, there's a doozy: Mom acting like it's a good thing I'm not skating.

"If it doesn't help," he says, "I'll put in a referral for a dietitian. Even a few pounds is too much for her to lose at this point."

"We'll make sure she eats," Dad says to Dr. Mu. "So will Gallagher," he says to me with a wink.

The medical student thanks me, wishes me good luck, and leaves.

Dr. Mu says the cardiac echo showed my heart's baseline functioning is normal. Other stand-out good news, "The survival rate for people with Hodgkin lymphoma is around 90 percent. It's an aggressive cancer, but it responds well to treatment." Therefore, I should "look at this whole thing as an inconvenience."

Speaking as someone who's experienced inconveniences—homework; my skate guy going on vacation when I need my blades sharpened—I can't see how three cycles of chemotherapy qualify as a mere inconvenience. It involves six infusions every two weeks over three months.

Mom asks Dr. Mu about *fertility preservation*. I imagine myself on a laboratory table with a fertility expert probing me. Then I imagine myself screaming, pushing out a baby. I wince at the thought.

Dad excuses himself to go to the men's room. His going would make the conversation less cringe for me and, I imagine, for him, but Mom calls him back. "Mason," she says, tilting her head and raising her brows. He returns to his seat.

The doctor says the odds of losing my fertility are pretty low. Mom says she doesn't think it's worth it for me to go through two weeks of hormone shots that, she fears, could increase my risk of getting other types of cancer when I get older.

She glues her eyes to mine, rests her hand on my shoulder, and says, "But it's your choice." She, of all people, knows about fertility treatments. She went through every type, so the story goes.

Being the offspring of a woman who wasn't ready for a child, I benefited from those treatments' failures.

"Even if the extracted eggs are still viable in ten or fifteen years," Dr. Mu says, "the odds of their transplantation turning into a pregnancy are low."

Throughout the discussion, Dad's face flushes and I cringe. My parents never even subjected me to "the talk," yet here we are, immersed in a physician-guided analysis of my future eggs' ability to connect with actual sperm.

Mom sighs.

I nudge her and say, "Let's cast this one to the universe. I'd rather start chemo immediately than waste time on a procedure with uninspiring results." Taking a pass on egg harvesting and extraction means no two-week delay in starting my treatments. I'm itching to get them over with and get this son-of-a-crud-bucket cancer out of me.

"If I'm infertile in the future," I say, "I'll adopt." Adopting's a win-win: I get to mother a child without having to push the kid out.

"We've made our decision?" Dr. Mu asks, sitting at his desk again.

"Yes," Mom and I say in unison.

"We'll schedule your first infusion then," Dr. Mu says. He hands Mom a folder, an "information packet."

She tells him Friday treatments would work best with her schedule. In response, he says, "Fridays it is. You may have to wait until next Friday, but I'll see if I can work my magic and get you in tomorrow." Part of that magic involves getting pulmonary function tests before I go home. One of the chemo drugs I'll receive can be harsh on the lungs.

AT 4 P.M. I sit in bed, reading a result of my *chemo, fertility preservation* internet search. It tells about a girl my age who harvested her eggs before getting a bone marrow transplant. They gave her hope for her future, something to strive for other than getting through her treatments. I get it. We make decisions based on our own unique cancers and insights. We're not in a one-size-fits-all situation. No choice is necessarily ideal, but each offers a crumb of control and a spark of possibility.

The baby odds are in my favor, I remind myself. I X-out the window. Besides, I already have something I'm looking forward to: finishing school and going to college.

Mom peeps into my room and says, "Can I come in?" As she walks toward me, her bob sways with a bounce my hair lacks. Her hair is straight and silky; mine is curly, only straight after a good flat-ironing. I scoot over, and she sits on the bed with me. "I imagine you're thinking about everything the doctor said. It's a lot to take in."

"You want to know what I'm thinking? Let me get through this cancer thing, and I'll worry about having kids later. Regardless of how I end up having them—if I decide to have them—it can't happen unless I'm alive. I don't want to give cancer a minute longer in my body, let alone two weeks."

She smiles. "Reasonable strategy. Have you thought about chemo, your hair, that kind of stuff?"

I run my fingers through my hair, which frizzed up from the humidity. Again. I flat-ironed and argon-oiled it twice today (before my tests and after I got home). As much as I complain about my hair, I hate the thought of losing it. It's part of who I am. "I wonder what my head looks like under this mop." Sweeping my hands across my skull, I conclude it's pretty round with no unusual protrusions. So far, so good.

"My friend knows a wig maker for actresses. She could make a custom one for you."

I crack my knuckles. "That's great, Mom, but please don't tell anyone else. And FYI, the doctor said everyone's hair responds differently. It could thin out without falling out."

She runs her fingers through my hair. "You must have been happy to hear again that your cancer is curable."

"Yeah."

She kisses my forehead. "I'll see you at supper. I have to get some work done."

There's a calmness about her, a shift from her initial reaction to my diagnosis. The softness of her voice; sitting, listening to me. No tears. Solid. Good vibes. As I requested.

She has shifted into lawyer mode, is in complete control. Like when she's on the phone, dealing with panicking clients. I've heard their voices echo from her office, worried, angry, heartbroken, or all of the above. Her shift gives me confidence and reinforces the credibility of what my father and my doctor told me: my cancer is curable. Confirming this, an internet search of *Hodgkin's lymphoma stage IIA*.

In this stage, the cancer is confined to the neck and chest, which describes my PET-CT. I don't have all the symptoms of Hodgkin's lymphoma (HL)—haven't had a fever, night sweats, or itchiness. Well, I'm a little itchy. While examining me, the doctor pointed out scratch marks on my hip.

What's this? Risk factors for HL include exposure to the Epstein-Barr virus, the culprit that causes mono. Some

Hodgkin tumors house EBV; therefore, the virus might contribute to some cases of HL.

Making out with Joao was literally the kiss of death. I wish I could go back in time and not kiss him. Then again, other girls kissed him and didn't get cancer. Let's face it: smooching is the springboard for baby-making. If kissing caused cancer, most of us wouldn't have been born. The human population would be on the Endangered Species list.

RANDOM FIND: other names for Hodgkin's lymphoma: Hodgkin lymphoma and Hodgkin or Hodgkin's disease. Make up your minds, people.

DISTURBING FIND: when people with my type of cancer die, it's usually the treatment, not their cancer, that gets them.

My eyes sting like a swarm of bees are taunting them into a good cry. I press hard against my tear ducts, a useless attempt to stop the flow. I'd given up competing, thinking I could actually enjoy life. Judging from what I've read, I'm still competing, all right. I'm in a competition for my life.

I haven't trained for this. I've never been in a competition I haven't trained for. I figured I could beat a curable but inconvenient cancer. Competing against a chemo treatment that can kill me? That's playing dirty.

I suck in a deep breath. Pursing my lips, I exhale slowly, and the tears stop flowing. I pat my face dry with a tissue, then grab a fresh one and blow my nose. Now that I've gathered my composure, a common-sense plan pops into my head:

I'll zero in on nutrition, germ awareness, and improving my repertoire with the Holy Ghost. I'll also focus on the positive information Dr. Mu told me: Treatments for HL have been modified over the years. As a result, they're less toxic to the heart and lungs than earlier treatments were. He and my nurse practitioner will monitor me closely for adverse reactions. If there's a problem, they'll modify my treatments.

My phone buzzes with a text from Will: *How's your marathon appointment going?*

Me: *It's going.*

Will: *I'll pick you up Monday morning for work and then take you to Gracie's lesson? Just confirming.*

I offered her a specific plan for Monday I can't renege on, so I confirm.

Game plan: Dr. Mu said I'm more apt to start chemo next Friday, a week from tomorrow. That gives me a decent window of time to draw up a plan for Gracie, secure her a coach (other than me), and invent an excuse for retracting my landscape-work offer to Will. I'll protect and hide my incisions, push through my Monday commitment, and possibly work through Thursday. I've been tired for a year—nothing new.

Will and I never discussed specific work hours, so he shouldn't get too mad if I bail on a full-time commitment. Landscaping work demands strength and stamina. Mine is compromised to begin with and will only get worse during chemo.

He texts me a thumbs-up.

The emoji of approval is a tiny Band-Aid on a potentially massive bleeder. Counting on me, at this moment in my life, is like counting on a parachute with a hole in it. My upcoming failure to work could be followed by a failure to follow through with my Gracie promises. Nathan might refuse to help me find Gracie a coach. My father might fail to find her a coach if Nathan doesn't come through. After a few treatments, I may be too sick to drive to the rink and watch Gracie for a few minutes, "just enough" for her to think I didn't forget her.

"Last search," I tell myself, opening a window I'd minimized earlier. It's a blog post written by a girl who received the same chemo I'm due for, the ABVD regimen. Each initial stands for a different type of chemo I'll receive. Dr. Mu blurted out the names during my appointment, but he may as well have been speaking Swahili. Anyway, the girl's neutrophils got so low she had to isolate. Without that specific type of white blood cell helping the immune system, she could die from a bacterial infection.

Positive thinking, Madz. The girl survived. But that must have been one hell of an "inconvenience." Another buzz diverts my attention to my phone.

Gallagher texts me for the first time ever. *Gracie's here. Shall I send her up or tell her you're sleeping?*

Send her up, thx. I jump out of bed, hurry to my mirror, and adjust my hair to cover my neck incision.

Gallagher: *thx?*

Me: *It's short for thank you:)*

Gallagher shows Gracie into my room. She hugs me hard, burrowing her head into my neck. Her chin digs into my biopsy incision, and her chest presses into my portacath. *Ouch.* The second we unhug, I sneak a peek in the mirror and readjust my hair.

"Will's working down the street, so I ran to your house when he wasn't looking." She's sweating, and her cheeks glow hot pink. "Were you crying?"

"It's my allergies." I pick a wilted dandelion from her hair.

"I put that there for decoration." Gracie takes the dandelion, and it flops over her fingers as she tries to tuck it over her ear again.

"You shouldn't run away from your brother. He'll worry

about you." I pick up my phone to text Will, only to find a text from him asking if Gracie's here.

I text him *Yes, and it's ok.*

Will: *Sorry. She took off while I was texting you. Tell her ten minutes—that's it.*

Me: *Ok.* I look up from my phone and tell Gracie. "You know, it's rude to look over someone's shoulder when they're texting."

"Yeah, but you're texting my brother, so it's okay."

"Not really." I head for the door. "Let's go outside."

We walk downstairs. Gracie peeks into Dad's office, where he's at his desk, peering at our souvenir from Dr. Mu, an information packet. Mom's hovering over his shoulder.

"Hi," Gracie says to them.

Dad's eyes hurdle his readers. "Hi."

Mom looks over hers. "Hello."

"They look really serious," Gracie says.

"They're working." I gently take her arm, nudging her along. "Come on."

I open the French doors in the kitchen, and we step onto the patio, where she rests the dandelion in a flowerpot and covers the end of its stem with soil. What better place to grow weeds than in the flowerpot?

She points to the gazebo. "Can we sit in there so the bees don't get us?"

"Of course. That's why it's there."

We screen ourselves in, and Gracie says the gazebo's our hive. I review what I'll teach her Monday and tell her to watch a few videos on my website. "While watching," I say, "pay attention to how I position my body—arm positions, hands, legs, feet, back."

"Okay," she says, texting.

She convinces Will to let her eat here and hang out with me while he goes on a date with Heels, a tidbit Gracie confirmed for me. I didn't invite Gracie to dinner, nor did I ask her to hang out with me, but that's what happened. Here's why I'm glad it did: Gracie reminds me I'm more than my diagnosis. She sees the healthy side of me, and that tells me it's good she's here, good I'm hanging out with a girl who's close to my age and living life outside the confines of a cancer diagnosis. It beats spending the day sleeping or scouring the internet for random information.

After eating, we head to my skating "closet," where Gracie tries on her favorite dresses. They're also my favorites. "Looks like they fit," I say. "If you need one for a test or competition, you know where to come."

Tears are like bees. A lot of times, they sting. They do now, when Gracie changes into her final pick, the red dress I wore for my salsa routine. I may not have enjoyed the pain and time demands of training, but I did enjoy performing.

Performing. Triggers the idea: *ice theater.* That would be perfect for Gracie. She'd have the opportunity to compete, make new friends, and participate in the skating world. Maybe even the SuperEdge skating world. All she'd have to do to try out is become a member of SuperEdge and pass her elementary skating tests.

"What do you think about working toward ice theater?"

"What's that? Do they put ice on a theater stage, and I put on a show?"

I explain what it is and what she'll have to do to get into it, including becoming a member of the SuperEdge Skating Club. I doubt she can afford the membership fee, but we'll cross that bridge when we get to it. She'll need two sponsors. Me (technically, still a member in good standing) and—here we go again—Nathan. Can't ask Lindsey. She and/or her mother might realize Gracie's the famous "screamer" from our old rink. They could put two and two together, with the help of Lindsey's former coach, and alert the board members of SuperEdge. This would ruin Gracie's chances of becoming a club member, making the ice-theater team, and, possibly, acquiring a suitable teacher. I'd never speak to Lindsey again.

"Can I still compete if I do ice theater?" Gracie asks.

"Yes, but you'll be competing with your ice-theater group. You'll like the coach. She's a sweet woman who's the spitting image of Mrs. Claus and always smells like gingerbread." It's the flavor of the tea she constantly sips. She's a walking, talking, skating room freshener.

"Okay, but can I still compete alone sometimes?" Gracie stands before the full-length mirror and turns left, right, and back-facing, looking over her shoulder at the mirror.

"Yes. Do what makes you happy. When it no longer does, you can stop."

Her eyes meet mine in the mirror. "Like you did."

Those words are little bugs gnawing at my gut. "Right." The word *stop* is so permanent; the thought of being forever detached from the ice, sad. "Or you can take a break or skate without competing. You have options."

"I was in a theater group for two years. Not on the ice. On a regular stage made of wood." She spreads her arms upward, kneels, and looks up to the ceiling as if asking God, "Why me?"

"Bravo!" I clap, more sure than ever she'll thrive in ice theater.

"I had to drop out. Will said I had to choose either skating or theater. 'Too expensive to do both.'" She says the last part with a spot-on impersonation of Will. "He won't let me do ice theater if it costs more than my usual skating. That's what he'll say."

"I'll talk to him when the time's right. We can't overwhelm him. Let's focus on preparing you for your elementary tests first." I hand her my favorite practice dress, which is nice enough to use as a test or competition dress. "For you."

Her eyes light up at the sight of the light-blue dress. Crystals dot the bodice, while chiffon adds soft, flowing lines to the skirt and three-quarter-length bell sleeves. "I'm going to look like an ice princess in this."

I fold the dress and put it in a gift bag. Mom says I hoard gift bags. I do, but only the pretty ones. "C'mon. Change into your clothes, and we'll watch a movie."

After she changes, we move to the home theater and sit in puffy, wide recliners. Gallagher surprises us with popcorn and root beer. I barely ate supper, so I throw a handful of buttery, salty heaven into my mouth and savor the smell and taste. I wash it down with the cold bottled soda, then press the recline button. Gracie follows my lead.

I click on the screen and navigate to *The Greatest Showman*.

WILL PICKS Gracie up at nine-thirty. Holding her gift bag, she runs into his truck, leaving him at the door with me.

"That won't happen again," he says. "Just say no if she pushes herself on you again."

My heart sinks into my stomach. "She didn't push herself

on me." She kind of did, but it worked out for all involved. Even my parents seemed relieved. For a while, with Gracie, I was a typical sixteen-year-old as opposed to a teenager thrust into a medical apocalypse.

"Yeah, she did." He sighs. "I don't want her burning you out too fast. I told her it's not appropriate for her to run to her temporary coach's house whenever she feels like it, but she has it in her head that you're her friend. Sorry."

"Maybe we are friends. And as my friend, maybe she won't yell when I give her a lesson Monday."

"That really bothered you, huh?"

"Yeah—I mean no." Truth: yes, it embarrassed me almost to death. "How did your date go?" I'm hoping it went horribly, explaining his early return.

Instead of answering me, he looks down.

"You smell nice," I say. "You must really like her if you put cologne on."

"One would think." His eyes find mine. They're even bigger and browner than I remember, with gold spots that twinkle as they catch the light from the door lamps. His cologne makes me want to wrap my arms around him and kiss him, but I feel the same way when he smells of freshly cut lawn and gasoline. "Thanks for helping me with my sister tonight. I can tell she had a good time."

Gracie waves to me, and I wave back. Hard to believe she's the same human siren who shrieked at the rink. "See you Monday?" I say to Will.

"Yeah." He looks down and turns. Shoulders slouched, hands in his pockets, he steps down the stairs and scuffs toward his truck. His shuffling steps tell me he's less thrilled than Gracie, who's still waving to me. A pang of sorrow jabs my conscience. I shouldn't have wished he had a bad time on his date. Working so hard and caring for his sister the way he does, he deserves to be happy.

I may have a cloud hanging over my head, but Will's eyes? His slouched shoulders? His heavy steps? They tell me he's got a cloud of his own to contend with.

SIXTEEN

After Gracie left my house last night, Mom told me Dr. Mu had scheduled my first chemo treatment for the following morning. Which is today, Friday. I woke up early, anxious to get my treatment over with. Each one I check off is a step closer to being cured and having an actual life. At the same time, I panicked because Dr. Mu threw me a loop: he said he'd rather I not skate, work with other kids, or landscape yet.

His reasons for the loop-throwing? He doesn't want me to catch an infection; he wants me to be as healthy as possible so I tolerate treatment. Also, he's not sure how my blood will react to my treatments, so he wants me to avoid the risk of getting injured or overly tired during them. He also said I'd be "quite tired" for several days following treatment.

"I'm used to being tired," I told him.

"You'll be more tired," he said.

I confirmed plans with Will. He expects me to teach

Gracie and work with him Monday, the one day I thought was feasible. I won't even be able to teach Gracie from the boards. Monday is also the day I intended to give him a game plan for Gracie's skating and an excuse for retracting my landscaping-work offer. The decent window of time I had to honor my promises has shrunk to a peephole. I've already stepped into the war zone, and there's no turning back until I'm cured.

Sitting in a cushiony recliner, I rest my eyes on a wall of floor-to-ceiling windows offering a view of Boston: the open sky above, the buildings squeezed into the hospital district below. The view is so massive that I feel like a shivering bird in a concrete tree, tethered to my nest by tubing.

"I guess we've learned to bring a sweater the next time," Mom says. She smiles at me, then looks at her computer and tackles her emails. She's taken her version of a leave of absence, working remotely as much as possible.

Candy, my infusion nurse, enters the room. She covers me with a warm blanket. "That'll get rid of those goosebumps," she says. Covered in a disposable gown, mask, and gloves, she washes my portacath off with antiseptic, punctures it with a needle bent at a right angle, and flushes the port with saline. It causes a fleeting alcoholish smell. She plugs an IV of normal saline into the port.

She gives me a small "test dose" of bleomycin to make sure I don't have a life-threatening reaction and can tolerate the prescribed dose. This bastard can hurt the lungs, but I try to imagine it as a cancer-killing beast.

"There are so many side effects to these chemo drugs," I say. "The manufacturers should list what they don't cause."

"Don't worry," she says. "We've got all sorts of tricks up our sleeves to keep you as comfortable as possible, and most people don't experience all the potential effects."

After a nail-biter of an hour, during which Mom and Candy watched me like sister hawks, I'm out of the life-threatening-reaction woods. For the moment. There's no guarantee future infusions won't affect me negatively.

Candy hands me a blue barf bag. "I'm hoping you won't need this, but just in case." I tuck it between my hip and the chair, and she hands me a medicine cup. In it are pre-chemo medications for fending off side effects: acetaminophen, diphenhydramine, a steroid, and a pill for nausea. I swallow them all at once.

Thirty minutes later, Candy sits beside my chair and delivers my "push meds" through a port on the IV tubing. Mom looks on with a furrowed brow as Candy pushes the first drug, doxorubicin, a red fluid nicknamed the Red Devil. (A brand name of it is Adriamycin, explaining the "A" in ABVD.) Throughout the five-minute push, she tells me about her puppy Frankie, a goldendoodle. I smile and nod, staring at the red solution entering the portacath, the portal to my insides.

"Don't be surprised if your pee looks red after this," Candy says.

"I'd rather that than the other things it can cause," I say. Nausea, vomiting, fatigue, diarrhea, hair loss, inflammation of the digestive tract, including the mouth, and low blood-cell counts. Or worse, it can harm heart muscle. This is why I got an EKG and cardiac echo prior to chemo and will get them in the future.

"Potential side effects aren't definite side effects," Candy says.

Already nauseous, I move the barf bag to my lap and grip it firmly.

The second push med is vinblastine. Many of its side effects are manageable and temporary, like the metallic taste in my mouth. What makes this sucker extra special is if it escapes the bloodstream, it causes considerable tissue damage and blistering.

Mom peeks up at me from her computer and says, "You okay? You look a little peaked."

I wrinkle my nose and shrug, not wanting to hear myself say "nauseous," which in and of itself sounds nauseating.

I'd planned to use this time to outline a plan for Gracie that I could give to Will. As I watch the cancer-killing chemical enter my port, acid rides up my throat and reality sinks in. There will be no outline. I can't concentrate on it while queasy from chemo and white-knuckled over potential assaults by other side effects. I write "Call Nathan" in my journal.

Mom eyes her phone. "Ugh, I'm sorry, Madz. I have to call work. I'll be right back."

I breathe in through my nose, blow it out through my mouth. I must tell Will ASAP I fudged up and can't work after all, so he can hire reliable help. Bailing on Gracie's lesson will be more painful. I need to secure a coach for her, one suitable for her learning style. Doing so is no longer about obligation. It's about her well-being. It's about Will's well-being. And mine.

Candy hangs the bleomycin, mixed in a 50 cc bag of normal saline. "This goes in over ten minutes," she says, setting the drip rate on the infusion machine.

I'd text Will my availability has changed, but then I'd have to explain how a week-long appointment morphs into a three-month-long appointment. He has enough going on with parenting Gracie and dealing with whatever it was that cast a gloomy cloud over him the last time we spoke. Being a no-nonsense guy with that kind of responsibility, he doesn't need excuses. He needs promises kept and honesty. Neither of which I can deliver unless I get creative. The solution: be partially honest and keep my promises by proxy.

Guess what? Lindsey texts. *I'm off the freaking waiting list! Nathan took me on as a student!!*

I'm shocked he did. She's coming off an injury and isn't skating at a level anywhere near his standards. I text her: *I'm happy you got what you wanted:)* This could close the door on Gracie. Nathan can only stretch himself so thin.

Ten minutes pass, and Candy hooks me up to dacarbazine. It doesn't just kill cancer; it can lower white blood cells and increase my risk for infection. Yay. Light-sensitive, this necessary evil comes cloaked in a brown bag and will make me sun-sensitive. I'll have to go into vampire mode. Two hundred and fifty milliliters will infuse over a half hour.

Fifteen minutes later, the queasies kick into high gear when a metallic taste locks onto my tongue again and sets off my hyperosmia. I can smell the weird taste. In fact, I can't escape the odor.

"Can you give me more anti-nausea medicine? This taste in my mouth . . ." I cringe.

"It's too soon," Candy says.

I hold the bag to my mouth and dry heave three consecutive times.

"Give her some gum," a child's voice says. It comes from a

corner across the room. A frail speck in her infusion chair, the girl can't be older than five or six. Her smile emanates a depth of kindness and understanding no child that young should be able to emanate. Clearly, she's a veteran of this war.

Candy draws my curtain. "I'll be right back." From beyond the curtain, she says, "Good idea, Chelsea."

Mom returns.

Gagging, I hand her my phone with Will's contact information pulled up and hurl exactly what I said he doesn't need: an excuse. "Text him and say I can't make it to work Monday. Tell him"—I retch. "Tell him I've come down with something and can't teach Gracie either." My journal drops on the floor as I puke.

Candy returns with a fresh barf bag. She takes the used one and hands me spearmint gum. It distracts my taste buds and nose enough to stop me from gagging. Fifteen minutes later, the infusion is complete, and I'm done with my first chemo treatment. Before disconnecting the IV, Candy "opens the line" of normal saline for a few minutes to flush my port and rehydrate me.

As Mom packs my journal into her tote bag, I draw my curtain back, hoping to wave to the little girl who helped me. She's asleep, but her mother waves to me. I smile and wave back.

"Let's go," Mom says, tucking her computer into her tote.

"I hate to get you in the middle of this, Mom, but I desperately need you to call or text Nathan when you get home. Tell him you're following up on what I asked him about Gracie. If you can't do it, remind Dad he promised me he'd help."

She hugs me. "I will, honey. Your father and I will take care of everything. Please don't worry about it. Focus on getting better."

"Okay, but if you or Dad can't call, you have to tell me so I can." How can I not worry about keeping my promises to Gracie and Will? Failing them, I'd fail myself. They'd lose all respect for me, and I'd lose them as friends. Ultimately, this monster of a disease could devour what's left of my dignity.

SEVENTEEN

I ride the chemo tilt-a-whirl for the next two and a half months, receiving my infusions every other Friday. The days vaporize into a montage of memories:

Me queasy, immune to the effects of antiemetics. Candy greeting me in her "hazmat" attire, her smile hidden by a mask but gleaming in her voice. Front-desk people greeting me like family. Celebrating my seventeenth birthday at home with Mom, Dad, and Gallagher.

In lieu of a gift, I asked my parents to buy Gracie a new pair of skates. Hers are broken down, mine are too small for her, and good ankle support is a must for skating. Gracie doesn't know about the new skates. They're not ready yet.

While some memories flash past as if swirling in a windstorm, others stick like paint on canvas. Such recollections are portraits of time with Chelsea, the six-year-old girl who told Candy to give me gum the first time I puked in the infusion room. Three more times I shared a chemo room with her. Like me, she'd lost touch with her friends. She'd homeschooled throughout most of kindergarten and missed first grade altogether because she was too sick to concentrate.

"I read books with my mother every day," she said. "And we play counting games. Mom calls it unschooling."

Once, we encouraged each other through simultaneous bouts of puking. On a better day, we had an "infusion-room picnic." During it, we nibbled on shortbread cookies, sipped apple juice, and watched me skate on a smart TV hanging from the ceiling. Her mother had found the video on the internet.

After watching it, Chelsea asked for my autograph, L to the O to the L, ha ha. Her mother handed me a picture of me that she'd printed off my social media account. I wrote, "To my best friend, Chelsea. You're the bravest girl I know. Thanks for helping me through my chemo. Love, Madz [heart]." At that moment, she really was my best friend. In fact, she was my only friend.

One day, when we were both not throwing up and not totally exhausted, our mothers took us to Fairies and Such Butterfly Garden. Going skating wasn't an option. It would have been too dangerous for her. A fall could trigger a fracture, a bleed, or a seizure.

Mom and Theresa sat on a bench while Chelsea and I walked around the butterfly garden. It was nice to see them chatting outside the hospital for a change, surrounded by life instead of pasty walls and the heavy stench of sickness. As Chelsea and I searched the garden for hidden fairies and butterflies, a butterfly landed on Chelsea's shoulder. She couldn't see it, so I placed my finger in front of its skinny legs, and it climbed on.

"Look," I said, holding it before her eyes. Wide open, they

fixed on it. The butterfly stayed there as if it knew she was taking in the details. As if it knew that she, of all people, appreciated the tiny details of its existence: curved wings outlined in black, filled in with shimmering midnight blue; its body narrow and featherlight, able to take off in a single bound and fly above anyone and anything effortlessly.

Most of the time, though, I stayed home. Gallagher watched over me while my parents worked, so the poor guy had to manage most of my nauseafests. The smell of breakfast nauseated me. The smell of lunch nauseated me. The smell of supper nauseated me. Hard candy didn't help. Fruit smoothies didn't help. Eventually, spearmint gum didn't help. It reminded me of chemo and made me more nauseous.

Only the aroma of fresh air and grass settled my stomach. So did the smell of falling rain. For those reasons and for the sake of my chemo-induced sun sensitivity, I spent a lot of time in the gazebo. When I wasn't too tired, I did homework for calculus and AP English in there to finish my online high school program. After meeting Chelsea, I realized time is too precious to shelve moments like empty glasses.

Mom let me take the twelve-week intensive courses because I was, and still am, on a daily quest to avoid germs determined to take advantage of my low neutrophils. Hanging out with "friends" could get me sick and delay my recovery, and *hel-lo*, I want a life ASAP. The online classes helped the weeks pass quickly but irritated my brain cells. Preferring as much sleep as possible, they protested and asked, *Why?* every time I worked on my homework.

I'm hoping Gallagher's latest smoothie recipe solves my energy crisis. He tried nine recipes before whipping up the highly palatable "Health Potion Number Ten" last week, a tangy treat made of frozen fruit, spinach, oat milk, and protein powder. It's one of the few foods that doesn't turn my stomach. Maybe now Gallagher will take a break.

His general routine has been he winks when our eyes meet but otherwise scurries about, cooking, cleaning, serving snacks when I study, covering me when I rest, and offering help or food or drink whenever I so much as flinch. I'm concerned he's become obsessed with waiting on me.

"Nothing bad will happen if you take a break, Gallagher," I told him recently.

"I'm on strike from breaks until you're better, my love."

Candy signals me into the infusion room.

"Let's go," Mom says.

Leaving the pediatric cancer clinic's waiting room, I glimpse at two patients who remind me of Chelsea. They're no more than six years old and are bald with lumps and scars marking their heads. I'm lucky. At least I lived sixteen years before going through this.

I enter the infusion room, sanitize my hands, and sit in a recliner. I adjust it so my legs are slightly elevated, then sanitize my hands again.

Mom shoulders her tote bag. "I'll be back after my conference call."

Five minutes later, Candy covers me with a lightweight blanket, hands me a barf bag, and slow-pushes doxorubicin. I turn my head and close my eyes, dreading what's to come. The ruby tide surges through my veins and crashes into my stomach, where the Red Devil flips it the double bird in spite of the new antiemetic Candy gave me. I sit up and hurl, thinking I'll never be able to look at red liquids again without hurling.

After throwing up, I take a sip of ginger ale, sigh, and

recline again, facing the window wall. Candy pushes in the vinblastine while I stare at the sky, imagining myself growing a set of wings and flying. I lift a tiny bottle of lemon essential oil to my nostrils and sniff, hoping this latest remedy of Mom's quells the queasiness that clips my wings.

One good thing, I no longer worry about who will coach Gracie. Nathan oversees her training. Mom called him, as I'd asked her, the Friday of my first treatment. However, my father had beaten her to it. That solved that dilemma.

My latest one? I fear Gracie and Will think I abandoned her, especially considering what Will said to me at UdderBuds Ice Creamery. I'm afraid to call them, afraid to let them in on my secret, afraid too much time has gone by to provide them with a reasonable excuse for not stopping by the rink to watch her skate. I've barely looked at my phone, scared of the texts I might see.

"Sounds like you're isolating yourself," Dr. Mu said during my clinic appointment. "Don't get me wrong. You need to be careful. But it's also important to have friends."

I told him my former best friend from SuperEdge hasn't bothered with me, neither have my other skating peers, and their snubbing me is for the best anyway. "Being with them could turn into a super-spreader event. One has chronically infected adenoids, another has a propensity for spreading mono, and who knows what all the others carry."

He suggested I speak with my psychologist, Harper. She was assigned to me shortly after my first treatment. Heeding Dr. Mu's advice, I told her, "Chelsea is my only real friend."

Her response? A head tilt, a furrowed brow, and the statement "Chelsea is your only real friend." It's called "verbal mirroring," a communication technique I learned in AP psych.

I took the bait for three reasons:

1. I had no one else to talk to due to burning the friend bridge.
2. I wanted to reward Harper for not overusing my name. (Usually, she attaches it to 95 percent of her statements.)
3. The session had a time limit. My only choice was to be a cooperative "mirror" myself and reflect.

"Chelsea and I haven't known each other long, but we're going through major crap together. We're both stuck in a bubble of treatments, tests, and clinic appointments. Life is going on without us. We don't have to explain to each other why we have no hair or, in my case, very little hair. We don't have to explain why we puke or look and feel washed out most days. For those reasons, I'm most comfortable with her."

"What's your favorite recent memory, Madz?" Harper asked. "As bad as your situation has been, you must have one."

I don't know if name-repeating is a therapeutic technique or a nervous habit, but if it's the former, the APA should rethink the method. So annoying. "Going to Fairies and Such Butterfly Garden with Chelsea."

Before that, my favorite recent memory was the time I landscaped with Will and Gracie. That was the last time I was outside the rink, the hospital, and my chemo-filled body, living a normal life.

Candy hangs the bleomycin, the potential lung-destroyer and fever-inducer. "Someone's in deep thought."

I smile. "Always. I have to distract myself from the demons raking my stomach."

"You're almost done with your treatments, so hang in there. You have a lot to look forward to." Leaving the room, she nods to—

What's this? O. M. G. I adjust my chair to sit upright, careful not to pull on the tubing my chemo infusion is dripping through.

"So," Nathan says, rubbing sanitizer into his hands, wearing a mask because this is my space and my face needs a mask break (at least until my nurse shows up again).

"So," I say, waving my hand toward the chair beside me.

"Nice beanie. Glad to see you haven't lost your affinity for Swarovski."

"I embellished it myself."

He sits. "I can't stay long. I have two hours to get Craig a birthday gift." Nathan and Craig have been together forever, so either Craig's a saint or Nathan isn't the cold-hearted ogre he comes across as.

"Thank you," I say.

"You already thanked me."

"Yeah, but not in person."

"Thank Lindsey. She's the one who took Gracie on as her volunteer project."

"I appreciate your help, but Gracie's not a project." Lindsey used the same description when she visited me during my second infusion, before my hair fell out. "And I did thank Lindsey. In a way. I told her she was doing a good thing helping Gracie." I said it after she confessed she was pissed about having to teach Gracie until she saw how cute her brother was.

"In case you don't know, Nathan, I didn't tell Lindsey that my parents and I were the ones who asked you to help with Gracie." I figured Lindsey would blame us for her having to teach the girl she refers to as *the screamer*. "Speaking of which, I'm surprised you chose Lindsey to teach Gracie. I thought you or another expert would coach her. Gracie's motor skills—"

"I assessed them and advised Lindsey accordingly."

"Her audio processing—"

"On it." He faces me again. "I gave her edge, three-turn, and spiral lessons twice a week, early in the morning, at that old rink in your town. She passed her elementary-maneuvers test Sunday." He puffs on his fingertips and rubs them against his chest.

"Nicely done. You *and* Gracie. I'm surprised Will paid for the extra ice time."

"I know the manager. He let us on for free. Hardly anyone skates there that early, and I wanted to clean up her technique before ice-theater tryouts. Change of subject. Joao's been asking for you. He says you blocked him last year."

"Long story."

"Oh, I know all about the kissing scam, trust me."

I doubt he's connected the mono I contracted last year to that scam. That was the real reason why I blocked Joao. "You didn't tell him, did you?"

"No. Your secret's safe with me. And it's safe with Lindsey. I told her she's not my student anymore if she tells anyone before you give the okay. She must have told you that. You guys were always together at SuperEdge."

"I haven't seen her since my second infusion." She and her mother dropped off a stuffed bear holding a Get Well balloon. "She came to keep me company, but I think she felt awkward." She scanned the room with a straight face and sanitized her hands *after* she left, not *before* she came in as Nathan did.

I got the impression Lindsey was afraid of catching my

cancer. She texted me twice in the two weeks after that to tell me how great she got along with Nathan and Will. To divorce myself from her annoying *Yay me!* texts, I was tempted to block her. I didn't want sympathy, but I didn't want people rubbing in how great their lives were when mine sucked.

Turns out I didn't need to block her. She took it upon herself to stop texting and calling me. What's more annoying, Lindsey wasn't honest about her relationship with Nathan. She was fresh off the injured list, not the typical candidate for Nathan's roster of students. It's no coincidence she started her "volunteer project" shortly after my father talked to Nathan about Gracie.

I take another sip of ginger ale. "I have a feeling you took Lindsey on as a student because she agreed to help you with Gracie."

"True. Lindsey was next in line on my waiting list, but she wasn't in prime condition. Her willingness to teach Gracie sealed the deal."

"And you're helping Gracie because you feel bad I have cancer."

"True. Ish. The main reason is"—he points at me. "Don't tell anyone this. I have a reputation to uphold."

"Okay."

"Your text brought back nice memories. They reminded me of an absolute treasure I once had in my life. Not just my brother but the whole experience. The Special Olympics, the camaraderie, the genuine love of skating, the love competitors had for each other and their coaches and trainers." He leans forward, and his eyes lose their usual squinty edge. "I don't have as much free time as I used to, but if I can help Gracie experience some of that joy, my brother is still here working his magic."

"Have you seen Gracie skate freestyle?"

"Twice. Once while guiding Lindsey through the first lesson and once at SuperEdge. Lindsey claimed to have a stomach bug, so I had to substitute for her."

"A stomach bug?"

"It was probably a reaction to all those green breath strips she ingests."

After the Joao incident, Lindsey developed a habit of sticking mint breath strips on her tongue. They mask the halitosis but tint her tongue green.

"What do you think about Gracie?" I ask.

When it comes to skating, I trust Nathan's judgment even though he's too tough sometimes. He's got a successful track record. In addition, a seriously good person has emerged from the rigid wall of uppitiness his coaching persona built.

"Her muscle tone, strength, and coordination are pretty good. I think she'll represent her skating level well in local competitions. She doesn't need to take the Special Olympics route; however, I told her brother she should consider volunteering at Special Olympics events. Working with those athletes will hone her sportsmanship. They set a good example. Long term, I'm thinking ice theater for her, given she's a drama queen."

"Exactly what I thought. I take it you've heard her scream?"

"I did, but I told her I wasn't impressed. I also told her if she loves skating, she won't scream anymore because it's not allowed on the ice, and she can't skate without ice."

I can imagine exactly how he said it, "how" being the key to

Nathan's overall success as a coach. So aloof it rebounds, burrowing into the deeply personal zone. I prefer Nathan's reason to Lindsey's regarding Gracie's cessation of screaming. When Lindsey visited me, she told me, "Gracie loves me. She never screamed once with me." The dig panged my gut.

How can a person drum up the gumption to make passive-aggressive comments to her sick best friend? The only answer I can come up with is I'm not her best friend anymore.

"Thank you, Nathan." My chin quivers as I hold back tears. I wish they'd go on strike. I blow them off with a couple of deep breaths.

"Why so sad? I thought this was your last treatment?"

"My last cycle. My final chemo infusion is in two weeks, but yeah. Almost done."

"What's going on? I won't leave until you tell me."

My eyes take on a life of their own and start leaking again. I was overdue for a self-pity party, never expected it to happen in front of Nathan. For the past three months, I've lived in a bubble, stuck like trapped gas in the intestines of life.

"Life's been going on without me," I tell him. "It's like every day I'm forced to miss a train to a magical place where I can do anything I want. I'm stuck in the same place every day. Not a geographical place. You know what I mean. I hate that about having cancer, the stuckness, and my prognosis is good. Someday I'll catch that train. But some people, one being a little girl I know"—I blow my nose—"have no hope of catching it. No hope, and they haven't even lived as long as I have. I hate that even more about cancer."

Every now and then, I get super sad about Chelsea.

"Life runs like time, Madz. It doesn't wait for anyone, no matter what we're doing or where we are. Whether we're learning, teaching, saving the world, or hanging out with a hot guy. So while you're forced to go through this." He waves toward the tubing plugged into my portacath. "Own the moment. Take it for what it is. I mean, you have no choice, right?"

"Right."

"This is what you've had to do to get better. If you don't fight through this last cycle and keep your eye on the prize, then you're not the girl I thought you were. Why do you think I took you on as a student in the first place? You certainly weren't the best jumper. I had no hope you'd ever land your doubles consistently, let alone land a quad."

"You still can't get over I suck at jumping. Even I was surprised you picked me over Lindsey to be your student." Before her growth spurt, when we first went to SuperEdge, her jumps were more consistent than mine.

"A lot more goes into a gold medal than landing jumps, and you don't suck at jumping. Most skaters never land a double axel, and even fewer land a quad toe loop. You can say you've landed both. It's just that your edges, gracefulness, and flexibility are exceptional. You could be a consistent gold medalist in ice dancing, and you know I have a thing for gold medals. But here's my point: jumps I thought you'd never land, you eventually landed because you fought for them. Other than the last time you skated, you'd brush yourself off, grow even more determined, and attack the next jump with a vengeance."

He stands. "Has Gracie texted you at all? She's skating tomorrow with Lindsey at the rickety rink."

"No, but you must already know that." Gracie and Will stopped texting me after my week-long appointment turned into a never-ending saga. On the Monday after my first treatment, the day I was supposed to teach Gracie but had to cancel, she rang my doorbell. I begged Gallagher to tell her I wasn't home. He shook his head, went outside, and walked her back to the house a couple of doors down, where Will was working. I melted down after that, crying off and on for an hour.

Harper specializes in cancer patients. I told her I have this thing in my head, one I've had since being diagnosed: I can't let people know I have cancer. If they find out, they'll think my death is inevitable, and I don't want those vibes sent out to the universe.

She asked me, "How are you so sure people will think that, Madz?"

Duh, lady, because that's what I always thought when I heard the word cancer. I didn't say it, didn't answer her at all, and she didn't push the issue.

Nathan says, "From what I hear—"

"Gracie and her brother think I dumped them."

"I told Lindsey to tell them it hurts you to be on the ice because you still love skating, and I won't take you back as a student."

Hmm. "Thanks?" I'd rather Nathan come out on top in the fake-excuse scenario if (1) it convinces Will and Gracie that my absence has nothing to do with them, and (2) the excuse doesn't have them thinking I'm at death's door. Yes, I have a curable condition, but some days, I'm so tired and pukey that I can't imagine doing anything but lying down in the gazebo.

Besides that, my infection-fighting capacity has red-zoned. In my eyes, strangers are germ zombies masquerading as humans. Another thing I've discussed with Harper.

I pull up my mask. Nathan's not a stranger, but living in the free world, he's been around a lot of them.

"I still think Will should text you," Nathan says. "I mean,

c'mon. What does he think? The good fairy plopped a free skating coach on his and his sister's doorstep?"

Will can't afford to pay over a hundred dollars an hour for Gracie's skating lessons. I'm sure Nathan's donating his time to the Gracie "Volunteer Project," an expression I plan to put a halt to.

Nathan gently squeezes my shoulder. "Text me how you're doing." He walks toward the door.

"Nathan."

He stops.

"Thank you. Really."

"My pleasure, doll." He blows me a masked kiss.

Candy hangs the final drug, dacarbazine, what I affectionately call the Pukinator. Like the Red Devil, it breaks through my nausea-medication barrier at the speed of light.

"We're at the home stretch," Candy says. "Are you excited?"

Clearly, she's focusing on the task at hand, not my tear-smeared face. I'm so over feeling like crap. I blot my nose and squeak out a weak "Totally. Yay." I'm happy I'm almost done but dread what's coming any minute. Besides that, I can't imagine having the strength to do my homework, let alone anything worthy of getting excited about. I'm lucky to have the strength to puke my guts up.

"I know you hate this one, Madz, but remember. It's almost over."

The Pukinator will go in over thirty minutes. It accentuates the essence of metal already latched on to my senses, making me hate it as much as I hate the Red Devil. I'd give anything for a whiff of freshly cut grass. Why hasn't anyone bottled that yet?

When Candy's done pushing, I hold my stomach, and she

hands me a new barf bag. I take a deep breath in through the nose, out through the mouth. It would have been a false alarm if Mom didn't come in with her lunch and trigger my hyperosmia.

Tuna. *Fish.* Previously canned, stewing in mayo. *Yecch.* Smells fishy. Fishy and dead. I hurl and, between heaves, try to force out the words, "dump the sandwich"—hurl—"far away"—hurl—"breath mints—take 'em before coming back." The Red Devil and Pukinator are angels compared to my hyperosmia lately.

Acid shoots up my throat. I'm a human volcano, erupting. It's never going to stop. "I can't"—hurl—"do this anymore."

Candy bins my puked-on blanket and covers my shirt with a blue disposable drop cloth.

Mom stares at me, cringing, slowly shaking her head. "Oh, honey, I'm—"

"The tuna"—dry heave. "It's still in here"—puke.

"I'm tossing it." She runs out of the room.

Moments seem like hours, and I'm convinced I'll drown in this vicious whirlpool. I want my life back, the one I had before my health went south. I'll take running around every minute of the day, energetic, skating, doing my off-ice training—pushing myself, being pushed—any day over this. I'd give anything to push my blades against the ice until I move so fast the cool air blows my hair. To spring into a jump and defy gravity, then stretch my arms out and touch down for a smooth landing and a deep, satisfying breath.

All of that's a dream, the opposite of what I'm doing: curling up in my recliner, retching into a blue barf bag. I cross into the panic zone and sit up, fearing I'll choke from the constant heaving before the nausea medicine I received earlier kicks in. If it kicks in.

Candy unleashes the saline, and I've never been more grateful for this portacath planted in my chest. Hydration is heavenly. She covers me with a fresh blanket and says, "Rest."

I follow her request because it requires no effort on my part. The Madz who flew across the ice? Long gone. I can't even walk across the room.

EIGHTEEN

Mom's voice floats into my ears, awakening me from my nap, but my eyes won't open. "I'm sorry I didn't go to your skating test," she says. "I'll regret that for the rest of my life."

You're just saying that because I have cancer. I'd say it, but who has the strength to talk? I could barely hold on to Mom's arm while she hauled me into the car, into the house, then into my bed.

I sink into my mattress, burying myself under an abundance of blankets. We complain all winter about the cold only to turn the AC down to "Arctic" in the summer.

She uncovers my head. "You took your final test after all the work you'd put into skating, and I missed it." Her fingertips gently sweep my cheek. "I'm proud of you. I was just too proud to say it before. I was too angry about your not following the path I thought you should've followed. But the truth is, you finished your commitment to skating with flying colors."

"Thank you," I croak. I click my shades open a crack, and the orange glow of sunset creeps in. Chemo ripped another day away from me.

Mom hands me my phone. "I think it's time you reconnect with the world. After you rest, of course. I bought Gallagher a new phone. He said you were the first person he'd text."

On cue, my phone buzzes with a text from him: *Cheer up, buttercup. Hope you're feeling better [praying hands] [four-leaf-clover]*

"Wow, Gallagher's using emojis now. Why do I find that funny?" I text back: *Getting there, TY [heart]*.

"Because Gallagher seems too sophisticated for such a thing." Mom sits on my bed again. "That ancient flip phone of his drove me crazy. He never texted. I had to call him for every little thing."

"He texted me once, when Gracie stopped by."

Gallagher: *TY?*

Me: *TY=thank you*

"Well, he never texted me. As much as your father and I love Gallagher's old-fashioned ways, we thought he needed a taste of the present."

"You wanted to face-call him every minute to check on me."

"Maybe."

Gallagher's making amazing progress. He group-texts Mom and me. I'm about to praise him when I see his message: *Gracie's here. [wide-eyed emoji] Shall I send her up or tell her you're sleeping?*

Mom and I goggle at each other. While I lie frozen in bed, stunned as if startled from a dead sleep, Mom's thumbs tap a mile a minute. Her text pops up on the group chat: *Tell her*

Madz has the flu and can't be around other people until she's better—doctor's orders.

I sit up. "I feel so bad."

"Me too. But we can't risk bringing in any germs from the outside. Unless . . ."

"No, not yet. She'd ask me a million questions, and I'm too tired. What if my answers scare her? What if the way I look scares her?"

This is the worst I've felt about withholding the truth from her. She may have bought Nathan's excuse for why I've steered clear of the rink. But how long can I make up excuses for refusing to see her in my home?

Did she leave? I text Gallagher.

His response: *Omg—Will came in, scolded her, and they left.*

Omg, Gallagher used the expression *Omg.* I text him a sad-face emoji.

Hiding from Will and Gracie hurts. I've moved on from worrying about them making assumptions about my life expectancy. Now I worry about how badly I've damaged my relationships with them by keeping mum about my illness. Just a few weeks more, and I'll make this up to them.

Gallagher appears in the doorway, panting. Hunched over, he holds the frame, his blazing cheeks lighting up his otherwise pale skin. Mom runs up to him. "What's wrong?"

He shakes his head. "I'm sorry. This is none of my business."

"At this point, we're all each other's business, Gallagher," Mom says. "Sit down. You're scaring me." She guides him to a chair and pulls down his mask. "Deep breath."

He takes a deep breath, pulls up his mask, and his eyes

creep from the floor to me. "I know you're weak." He looks at Mom. "I know she can't afford to pick up an infection, but we have masks, hand sanitizer, and lots of space for social distancing." He eyes me. "And I understand that whether or not you tell people you're sick is your choice."

"I know the *but* that's coming, Gallagher. You don't have to say it." What little blood I have pulsing through my veins finds its way to my throbbing head.

"I think I do have to say it. I think you need to hear the words, my love." He asks Mom, "Can I?"

She nods and sits on my bed.

"Gracie admires you," Gallagher says to me. "I'll go so far as to say she counts on you. More so as a friend than as a skating coach."

"I know."

"You didn't plan on her coming around, but she did. And you enjoyed yourself. Eating popcorn, watching a movie, giving her a grand tour of your skating closet. I'd never seen anything like it all the time I've lived here."

"It wasn't that bad, Gallagher, was it?" Mom says.

"No, of course not, but Madzy's life has been extremely regimented. That word you use in figure skating. Freestyle, is it?"

Mom and I nod.

He looks at Mom. "When Gracie visited, Madzy freestyled through her time instead of conforming to a schedule. But I'm not here to judge. What I want to say is . . ."

"It's okay, Gallagher," Mom says.

He straightens his back, and his blue eyes twinkle through a scolding squint. "It's just plain cruel to lie to that girl and her brother, and I have never thought of anyone in this family as cruel."

He stands, paces by the windows, and peeks through the curtains.

"Are they still out there?" I ask.

"No."

"Gallagher?"

"Yes, love." He says it with the enthusiasm of a competition loser.

"I need three weeks. That's it. A week after my last treatment, sooner if I have the energy." Chemo sucks the life out of me for days, rendering zilch desire to do anything, much less explain my illness, germ phobia, and hyperosmia.

Gallagher sighs. "I'll fix something to eat, something easy on your stomach."

"Vanilla ice cream is good enough." I bury my head under my covers again. "Make sure he heard me, Mom. My throat is still irritated, and I'm Health Potioned out."

The image of Lindsey sanitizing her hands after she left my infusion room, not before, pops into my head. Ugh, and those dwindling, annoying "freaking" texts of hers . . . If that's how all my friends would have acted, I'm glad I self-protected by not telling them about my illness. Lindsey bruised my heart.

The unfortunate twist, I've multiplied that single bruise into a throbbing constellation by shutting out Will and Gracie.

"I have an idea," Mom says, uncovering my head. "If you feel better tomorrow, how about we go for a ride? You need fresh air. You need to see the light of day."

At the moment, getting out of bed equates to climbing Mount Everest. I doubt a single night's rest can restore my lost energy. I pull the covers back over my head and say, "If I'm not too tired, okay."

NINETEEN

The crystals on my chandelier sparkle and dance in the morning sun. I wish I were one of those sparkles, free of this headache that started during last night's nightmare:

The rink was warmer than usual; the air, thick and damp. I expected the ice to be soft, but it was hard like when I tested. Moving faster with each stroke, I thought, *Good, the hard ice will make up for the thick, wet air.* Nathan hollered at me to enter a camel spin from a spiral, a move I can easily do outside this nightmare. As I crossed over in the corner of the rink, my edges lost their grip.

Struggling to balance, I passed Nathan and said, "I need my blades sharpened."

"Shut up and spiral into a camel spin," he said.

I pushed off into an arabesque spiral and tried to hold the dull edge, but it refused to grip the ice. My head ached. I spotted Will in the bleachers, throwing up his arms and shaking his head.

I thought, *Why is it bothering him that I'm slipping off my edge? Doesn't he understand I have dull blades and a headache?*

Gracie sat next to him, pointing at me, crying, and Mom shook her head, annoyed I didn't keep my sharpening appointment. Dad clapped and smiled, saying, "Good job, Madz."

My shoulders overcompensated on the curve into the spin. I was too weak to adjust but straightened my skating knee anyway. I kept spinning and spinning and spinning, unable to check out of it. My stomach whirled with the twirling, nauseating me, and my headache intensified. I fought against falling as I traveled across the ice, heading for the boards. Fearing I may bump my head on them, I tightened my core, bent my skating leg, and struggled to check out of the spin. Instead of checking out, I woke up from the dream sweating, my heart thumping hard against my chest; my brain throbbing, determined to bust through my skull.

I take two acetaminophens and throw on my clothes. I held my dinner down last night, my heart's no longer rattling my rib cage, and I'm determined to live some semblance of life today by going for a ride.

I open my makeup case and get to work. I glue on false lashes, conceal dark circles under my eyes, and brush a smidge of pink blush on my cheeks. For a final touch, I dab on pink lip gloss. There it is: a fake healthy glow. Dr. Mu said my last scan confirmed the cancer has backed off, and I won't need radiation. A final round of chemo and a few months of recovery stand between my fake healthy glow and my real one.

I pull my pink crystal-embellished beanie over my wig. WeatherAnt is calling for a tropical storm later today, and the last thing I need is my fake mop of "real hair" to pop off my head and catch the wind like a flying squirrel. Also, I feel less imposterish wearing the beanie. It covers half of the donor's hair, so I'm only being half deceptive about the locks being my own.

My hair didn't fall out all at once or completely, but when it got to the point where I could guess how many hairs were left on my head using an imaginary grid, I shaved it off. This removed the displeasure of waking up every morning to clumps of hair clinging to my pillow, spewed out by my chemo-poisoned follicles. It also ended shower-drain clogs.

"Cute," Mom says, adjusting the back of my beanie, finger-combing the back of my wig.

"Acceptable," I say, facing the mirror. "Do I look totally nuts wearing a beanie in August?"

"It's cotton, so no. You're a teenager making a fashion statement. How about after our ride, we stop at that cute bistro in Melrose to get a croissant?"

"Let's do it." My response is grounded in my consistent ability to tolerate a freshly baked croissant. As she drives, I meditate on growing an appetite. It's the least I can do for her after how she's catered to me, working out her schedule so she can spend time with me *and* get through her cases.

She told me she's gotten better at delegating authority at work, and the feat has "mitigated" her control issues. I believe it. She no longer measures her wine; she dumps it into her glass (to the same level as when she measured it). When she drinks. She cut down to twice a month. She says she's been too busy to indulge, which means she's been too busy to relax. That's a shame because she was already too busy, in general, before I got sick. I can only conclude that she can't relax because of me.

Mom rolls down the windows, I recline my seat, and we start our jaunt around town. I'm confined to the car, but at least the scenery changes. Yawning, sluggish from yesterday's chemo, I perk up when we cruise past my hometown's "rickety rink," as Nathan calls it.

"Gracie has a lesson this morning," I say. "Nathan told me Lindsey teaches her every Saturday morning."

"I'd say let's go in, but it's Saturday," Mom says. "The rink will be crazy busy. We can't risk you picking up an infection."

"I'll watch her through the window of the door separating the rink from the lobby." My stealthy appearance will allow me to assure Gracie, in the future, that I made an effort to watch her during our time apart.

I relay critical tidbits of information I gathered before leaving the house. "Group lessons don't start until ten a.m., and hockey has already ended. This freestyle session should be slow because there's a competition in Peabody."

"Peabody?"

"It's a non-qualifying competition."

We pass Will's truck in the parking lot. My heart beats faster, intensifying the throbbing in my head.

"I found a flyer in the mailbox," Mom says. "Gallagher saw Gracie put it in there. Will's advertising fall cleanup and that he added snowplowing to his winter services. Already thinking ahead for the winter. He's a hard-working young man; I'll give him that."

I put my mask on and enter the lobby. A guy in the office to my right waves. I wave and then look into the rink through a door window. Can't see anyone, so I creep into the frigid, near-dead rink, stand beside the bleachers, and peek over them. Hoping to clear my head, I pull down my mask. The crisp, cool air is a welcome break from the stuffy, masked air.

Will's at the far end of the rink, sitting on the bleachers.

Lindsey stands on the ice at the same end, talking to Gracie, watching her as she skates off and stops near the center. "This Is Me" plays, and Gracie begins her program. Lightheaded, I inhale a deep breath, blow it out, and focus on the technical aspect of Gracie's skating.

She starts off holding her arms up, but as she pushes through the program, attempting specific maneuvers—three-turns, a mohawk—her arms fly all over the place. I think concentrating on the choreography takes her mind off technique, but that can be fixed once she's gotten the program down. She falls on a waltz jump-toe loop combination.

"Get up," Lindsey hollers, shaking her head.

Gracie has the same look on her face as when she yelled during our lesson. I pull my mask over my nose and mouth again, wanting to hide from what's coming, and I cover my ears. She stands, pauses for a few seconds, then resumes skating, finishing her routine with an attempted camel spin and a traveling scratch spin. I'm proud of her. It doesn't matter that she fudged up or traveled during her spin. She didn't scream, and she completed her program despite falling and Lindsey's annoying *Get up!*

Just as I pull down my mask to blow my runny nose, Gracie looks in my direction. I duck, turn, and *Boom!* My eyes have a nuclear-powered clashing with Joao's. I gasp and pull up my mask.

"What, I scare you now?"

"Hey. How have you been?" A stranger's voice just came out of my mouth; I hope it sufficiently faked casualness. He's thrown a wedge in my plan to observe Gracie in a minimally infectious space.

He moves in for a hug. I hold my breath to prevent his

exhaled germs from migrating through my mask and entering my nostrils. A few seconds later, I push away from him, exhale, and suck in a deep breath, hungry for air. His smile levels, giving him a serious look.

"I've been asking for you, but Nathan keeps saying the same thing, 'Madz is Madz.' And you know Nathan. I don't push the issue. How are you?"

I'd be better if he'd break eye contact. "I'm great. Like, really great, Joao. Thank you. Thank you for caring to ask." I break his grip on my gaze and spot Will at the boards, talking to Lindsey. She leans toward him, whacks his arm, and giggles, her typical flirting technique. He smiles at her. Hello, people. Gracie needs a coach, not a disgusting display of cliché.

Lindsey has officially hijacked my life, and a jerk named Hodgkin Lymphoma helped.

Shivering, I cross my arms.

"Are you okay?" Joao asks, reining in my attention.

"Yeah. Uh,' what are you doing here? Shouldn't you be training?"

He holds open the glass door to the café, a term I use loosely. On a positive note, the room has heat. "Why are you acting so weird?"

"I'm not—"

"And why the mask? Last I checked, the pandemic was over."

"There's a strong chance black mold grows in this place. It's so old and damp in here. You should put one on too."

He scans me up and down, squinting, studying me like I'm a curious piece of artwork. "You're sick. Maybe we're not friends anymore, and maybe I was a jerk. But I can tell, and I care."

I sit at a table. "You think I'm sick." Harper's not the only one who can verbally mirror. I cross my arms and legs as tightly as possible to fight off the feral goosebumps pecking at my body. Joao sits on the other side of the table. He leans forward, too close to my personal space, so I push my chair back to a safe distance.

"Before you left the rink," he says, "I didn't think you looked right. I mean, you were—are—still pretty and everything, but you looked tired and a little too skinny. You lost your butt."

"Only you would determine the status of my health by the appearance of my ass."

"It's a skill."

My jaw stiffens as I try to prevent my teeth from chattering. I scrunch into my knotted arms and legs to fend off another pack of rabid goosebumps. "Why are you here and not at SuperEdge? You should be training for sectionals."

"This is my day off, and I'm taking over for Lindsey. She's almost done with her volunteer commitment, and I need a good one for my Harvard application. Nathan thought I should check out Gracie during one of her lessons with Lindsey before I take over. Lindsey's gonna give me a report on where we're at with Gracie's training. Her strengths and weaknesses, goals, learning style, and all that."

"She's not a project." I glance at the glass door. A portion of the rink is visible, but I can't see Gracie.

Joao gently sweeps his finger under my chin, prompting me to look at him. "Earth to Madz, what are you talking about?"

"I'm talking about—I mean, Gracie's not a project. She's not a volunteer commitment. She's a girl who loves skating and wants to learn. She's hard on herself and her coaches because she cares so much." I stand, determined to leave before I puke. The room dims as blood rushes from my head to my feet.

He stands and approaches me. As he moves closer, I back up to the wall. "Distance yourself." The words slipped from my mouth, outing me as a visiting alien, fearful of humans. Here I am, the girl who doesn't want her friends feeling awkward around her, churning out awkwardness.

His eyes move from mine to my shoulder. "What's this?" Frowning, he touches my hair-that's-not-really-my-hair.

I take a deep breath and focus on my goal, as I've trained to do. Only instead of nailing a skating routine, I must hold myself together. It's not happening. Two obstacles threaten my performance: his proximity and my shivering. I'm unraveling.

Short of breath, I pull down my mask. Catching more air has taken priority over catching an infection, which I may have already done. I turn my head away from him, toward the door. My eyes clash with Will's. They dart back to Joao.

He rubs my arm. "You look pretty. The hair, everything. It's just, I know your waves and curls, and they're not usually so . . . tame."

My eyes skip back to the door. Will's gone. Was I hallucinating? I'm nauseous *and* lightheaded *and* shivering now. "You can't tell anyone. Please."

"I won't. Did I ever tell anyone about our encounter at second base?"

"Ugh, stop. Forget that happened, will you?" With firm eye contact, I tell him, "You gave me mono. You should know that. And mono made me miserable."

He steps back. "You have mono?"

"No. You gave it to me last year."

"You didn't get it from me. I've been fine. Maybe you got it from one of the girls I kissed. When you kissed me, you kissed everyone I kissed before you." He smirks.

I roll my eyes. "Let's not go there."

His face grows serious.

I have to get out of here.

"What do you have?" he asks.

"Lymphoma." Blood rushes through my chest like I'm jetting down the highest point of a roller coaster. A warm wave of bile rolls up my throat. I feel weird. I'm losing control of my body in a . . . weird way.

"Lymphoma is cancer, Madz. Should I donate my bone marrow? I will, you know."

"My counts are stable. I mean, I can get an infection. Can't get . . . too close." *Is this chemo brain?* "You're sweet to offer." Gracie's famous yelp echoes from beyond the café doors. Am I hallucinating?

"Shit," Joao says. "I thought Nathan got her to stop that."

My phone buzzes with a text from Mom: *Are you ok? Come back to the car [prayer hands]*

"Will you unblock me so I can text you? To check on you," Joao says. "I still consider you a friend, no matter what happened."

"I'll unblock you if you promise not to tell anyone. About me. Lindsey knows, but she's sworn to secrecy too."

"Lindsey kept a secret?"

I know, right? I want to say it, but my throat's too busy holding down stomach contents. The urges to bolt like Cinderella at midnight and to puke have equalized. "I have to go."

He hugs me again. Before I can take a deep breath and hold

it. When I pull away, he holds me a second longer and says, "You're hot."

"C'mon, Jo—"

"No. Your cheek is hot."

I push him away. "I guess you have that effect on me." Any blood flowing to my brain has officially clogged, causing me to sway. Lights flicker and dim, the ones in my head, not the rink. "Bye."

Bolting through the café doors, I keep my head down and aim for the lobby door. The Zamboni hums as I pass work boots on my way out. Will's? My fading hearing picks up unintelligible chatter. No time to check if the muffled voice belongs to the boot-wearer. I push the door, run through the lobby, push the entrance door, and run to the car.

Shivering, I clutch my stomach as it joggles through a massive pocket of gastric turbulence. I open the car door, shut it behind me, and puke all over the floor.

"God, help us," Mom's muffled voice says. She accelerates so hard I fall back into the seat. *Shut off the AC.* The words die behind my chattering teeth.

In a blink, medical personnel lift me out of a wheelchair I don't remember getting into. They put me on a stretcher, and I contract into one bodily ball of shivers.

I OPEN my eyes to Mom. Wrapped in a yellow paper—a mask and a yellow disposable gown—she's a glowing orb hovering over my bed. "Sun," I say. She knits her brows together and rests her gloved hand on my forehead, indicating she doesn't get the joke.

A galaxy gleams where the ceiling should be, and I think, *Cool, I'm in space, closer to Heaven. Now I don't have to travel so far with all this weight on my chest.*

An X-ray tech wheels in a machine, sucking me out of my cosmic journey. After the chest X-ray, another yellow-paper-wrapped humanoid walks in. He adjusts the drip rate on my IV pump and says, "I need to swab you for flu, covid, that kind of stuff. Okay?"

As if I have a choice.

Nurse Nosepoker sticks a swab up my nostril and swirls the thing. He repeats the process with a fresh swab, this time shoving it almost into my brain. "How's the nausea? I gave you medicine for it earlier." He pulls out the swab.

"No more nausea." My reward for saying that? Throat culture. Because why not poke the hornet's nest and see if we can get Madz to puke again? I don't, but . . .

Coughing attack. Is a piece of lint stuck in my airway? A fiber from the throat-culture swab? I can't clear it. The coughing makes me retch, and the retching stuffs my nose, suffocating me. The nurse attaches a mist-blowing mask to my face.

"It will help your cough," he says.

Later, the ER doctor says the strep, covid, and flu tests are negative, but I have "a touch of pneumonia."

Worn out, waiting to be transferred to a regular hospital room, I fall asleep under the fake galaxy.

TWENTY

After five days in the hospital, I'm hydrated and fever-free. If that was a touch of pneumonia, I'd hate to get a full-on whack. Lucky for me, my counts were good enough to work with the IV antibiotics and kick the nasty microbes out of my lungs. The doctor thinks I handled the infection well because I skated so much in the past.

"You have strong lungs," he said, "and you're a fighter. Once a competitor, always a competitor." He also said the pneumonia wasn't bad enough to cause such intense symptoms. My chemo drug bleomycin may have contributed to them. For that reason, I won't receive it during my final round of chemo.

Mom returns my previously confiscated cell phone and gives me a masked kiss on my forehead. "I have to go to work, but your father will be here within the hour."

Alone in my room, I scan my texts and discover why she confiscated my phone. Gracie messaged me saying she cried when she found out I was at the rink and didn't say hi to her.

Will texted five days ago: *You lied about not letting down my sister, and today you didn't wave to her because you were too busy flirting with her new coach. Who was supposed to be watching her skate, not playing with your hair. Then, you ignored me when I asked if I could talk to you? Sad. For a while, I thought you were a nice person.*

I drop my phone on the bed and close my eyes. Will has some nerve lecturing me after he engaged with Lindsey's aggressive flirting during Gracie's lesson.

I set his sister up with a good skating regimen, and they moved on. While I'm stuck in Limbo with clipped wings, they're spreading theirs, progressing in life. Instead of picking up on cues indicating I was sick, he assumed the worst. He showed me no pity.

Congratulations, Madz, you got what you wanted: no pity. Too bad you left a flaming disaster in your wake.

Determined to heal the hurt I've inflicted upon Gracie, I muster the nerve to text her: *I have pneumonia. Got super sick. Sorry I didn't get to say hi. [Waving-hand emoji] [pink flower emoji]*

Five days ago, Gallagher told her I had the flu. Bad karma came whirling around in a flamboyant 180 and gave me pneumonia. He'd better stop making up illnesses for me lest they boomerang again.

I unblock Joao, sticking to the promise I made to him. A text of concern will be a welcome addition to my message box. No scolding me, no rubbing in (à la Lindsey) how great things are at SuperEdge.

Gracie texts: *Will says if you had pneumonia, why did you go to the rink and flirt with Joao? Don't tell him I told you he said that!!!*

Me: *I didn't flirt with Joao, but I'm surprised Will noticed us given he and Lindsey were flirting. Don't tell him I said that.*

Gracie: *She flirted with him. He was polite to her because she gave me lessons. Duh.*

After a moment, she sends me another text: *Do you know Lindsey? Why is her tongue green? It scares me but I don't say anything because I need a coach.*

Candy peeks into my room for another "door visit." She did the same when she was "in the neighborhood" a couple of days ago.

"Nice to see you in normal clothes again," she says. "When are you leaving?"

"In a little while. I can't wait to get out of here. I'm tired of looking at the same walls."

"Good. That tells me you definitely are better. Stay that way so I can see you next week for your last treatment, alright?"

I give her the thumbs-up, and she leaves.

I text Gracie: *Lindsey and I were best friends when I skated at SuperEdge. Her tongue is green from the mints she eats. I assume they're working, as evidenced by the absence of breath comments.*

Gracie: *Mints? That's a relief. I thought she was part alien [space-ship emoji]*

I put my mask on and peek down the hall. The nurse taking care of me on this floor passes by.

"Can I go for a walk?" I ask her.

"Sure, but don't go too far. The doctor should be here within the hour with your discharge instructions."

Judging from what I hear and smell in the hallway, I'm swimming in a Sea of Germs. God knows what these kids are coughing up and pooping out. However, the aromatic undertones of disinfectant tell me the staff is on top of the situation.

The nurse waves to me before entering a room. An X-ray tech passes me, pushing her machine. A PCA walks by, pushing a vital-signs machine. A lunch lady carries a tray into a room after parking her cart. Navigating the hallways of a hospital is similar to navigating the skating rink. Everyone's focused on their routine; you just have to stay out of each other's way. Walking this hall, I'm like a new skater, clinging to the sideboards.

"Hello, Chelsea," a voice in a room says.

This isn't the chemo suite, and a hospital can have more than one patient named Chelsea. I doubt any are as sick as mine. She has brain tumors, and her cancer spread to other parts. (Her mother told mine when we went to the butterfly garden.) A nurse leaves the room the familiar greeting escaped from. I hope the patient isn't my Chelsea. If she's here, her condition is deteriorating.

I peek into the room and wilt. It's her. She's wearing a pink beanie with an iron-on butterfly embellished with crystals. I made it for her to match mine. She looks sicker than usual. Her eyes, which meet mine, have sunken into gray halos, and she's ghostly pale.

"Madz." She pats her bed with a single weak pat, and I sit beside her.

"Do you want this?" I pick up a stuffed bumble bee from her bedside table and tap her nose with it. "Bzzz." I tuck it between her arm and torso.

The corners of her lips go up. "I like bees that don't sting."

I hold her cup of juice to her mouth, put the straw between her lips, and she takes a sip.

She closes her eyes. Cancer's exhausting, and her exhaustion must be a thousand times worse than the worst exhaustion I've felt throughout my illness. Her cheeks have swelled from steroids, and her small, pouty lips blend in with the rest of her skin. She looks like a cherub whose pink glow flickered out. She says something, but I can't hear her.

"What did you say?" I lean forward, my ear close to her lips.

"You're my friend."

I expected a warm puff on my ear when she spoke, but my ear remains cool; the air around it, unstirred. Even her breath is exhausted.

I gently squeeze her hand. "I am your friend. Always." I whisper in her ear, "Maybe I'll have a surprise for you the next time I see you."

She smiles but doesn't open her eyes. "I like surprises." Her hand twitches in mine like she's trying to squeeze my fingers, but her fingers are too tired.

"See you soon." I pull down my mask, kiss her forehead, and pull my mask up again, confident I'm safe. I've been tested up the ying yang for viruses and pumped up with hardcore "antibeez," my nurse's nickname for antibiotics. On my way out of the room, I run into Chelsea's mother. She gasps.

"It's Madz. I was saying hello to Chelsea."

"Hi," Theresa says. "I know it's you; you just startled me. I'd hug you, but—"

"I know. Social distancing."

"I'm so sick of that expression, aren't you? I spoke with your mother the other day. I'm glad you're doing better."

"We're taking her now," a nurse says to Theresa.

I assume Chelsea's going for a scan. Here, lab and X-ray

techs come to us, and her body doesn't look like it could take one more drop of chemo or one more zap of radiation. I head out of her room and back to mine, where I let loose an abundance of tears. The air was so heavy in Chelsea's room it hurt. It weighed heavier on my chest than pneumonia had. Chelsea's life is hanging on by a frayed thread, and I had the nerve to think it was the end of the world if people knew I had cancer, a kind that's actually curable.

I've never missed feeling normal more. I've never missed my old life as much as I do now. And I miss my skates. I miss the ice. Who cares about triples and quads? I'd be happy to spread my arms out like wings and fly across the ice in a simple spiral—cool air against my face, beautiful music playing. I'm so lucky I know how good that feels and how good feeling good feels. The memory may have faded, but it's there. That's more than Chelsea ever got. She's been sick her whole life.

So unfair.

Harper knocks on my door. "Do you want to talk, Madz? I'd just left one of my patient's rooms when I noticed you leaving Chelsea's looking a little sad."

I'd rather not get into a discussion when I'm inches away from breaking out of here, but I don't want to be rude. At least she cared enough to ask. "As I told you before, Chelsea's been my only friend these past few months. She's a sweetie."

"She's gotten sicker, huh?"

"Yeah."

"How does that make you feel?"

C'mon, lady, be original. An obvious wreck deserves more than generic psychobabble. "Not good, that's for sure." But since she asked . . . "It makes me sad. And it makes me angry that Chelsea is so young and weak and sick, stuck in a hospital while life's going on without her. I'd like to find out why people can go into space and robots can land on Mars, but no one can fix Chelsea's cancer. It's inexcusable." My break from crying has ended.

She hands me a tissue. "Sometimes it's worse watching someone else going through it."

"She's so young."

"She loves to watch figure skating. In fact, she showed me a video of you skating. She's very proud that you're her friend. She and her mother gave me permission to say something to you, Madz. So did your mother. You ready?"

I nod, wary of what's coming.

"Chelsea has a last wish. She said it would make her really happy."

I know where this conversation is going. "She can't skate in her condition. Let's put her in a wheelchair and take her to the butterfly garden again."

"She was very clear. She wants to skate with you. You're right about her inability to skate. However, she can put on a pair of skates and hold your hand. If we can figure out a way to prop her up. I know you've been weaker than usual yourself."

I can barely hold myself up, let alone Chelsea. "The rink has a few ice walkers. Kind of like the walkers old people use, only these are made for the ice."

"You can try it, but someone will still have to spot her, and when I say 'spot,' I mean hold her up. Her cancer is in her bones now. If she falls, they'll break, and the last thing she needs is more pain. Do you know a skater at the rink who's strong enough to hold her steady?"

Chelsea is in no condition to go on the ice. I want to grant her wish, but unless we push her around the ice in a wheelchair, I'm not sure how this will work.

"Madz, I'd never ask if this weren't such a special case. I'd truly appreciate your help."

"Let me ask around. When do you need to know by?"

"Yesterday? I know—ouch, right? She's very sick, Madz, but she's insisting she wants to skate with you. I believe that's why she's hanging on. Her mother is willing to take the risk because, well, you can imagine. She's hoping Chelsea can have one more happy, normal moment before she dies."

Is it normal for a shrink to get into this with a teenage cancer patient?

"Your expression tells me you're hesitant about this, Madz. No pressure. And Madz. Hear me out. This is very important. Chelsea's cancer is much different from yours. You're going to be fine." She pauses. "You look like you're thinking. May I ask of what?"

"I'm thinking . . ." *Stop saying my name every two seconds. How's that for a thought?* "I can figure out the logistics of getting Chelsea on the ice with me. If that's all I have to do to make her wish come true, I'm in." I shake my head, trying to shake off another wave of sorrow and tears. "So. Not. Fair. She's six." I blot my eyes and nose.

Who's in charge of this show down here? Where's God? Cancer should not afflict children.

To think I was embarrassed by Gracie's screaming and shuddered at the thought of being near it. I'd give anything for Chelsea to have the strength to yell out in frustration. I hope Gracie never loses that spark of fury, a sign she's alive and strong. "I'm sorry. I don't know why I can't stop weeping."

Harper springs an ocular leak herself by the window. She picks up a full box of tissues, pulls one out, and blots her eyes before offering me the box. I pull out a fresh sheet to replace the one disintegrating in my hand.

"It's okay to be sad," she says. "Why wouldn't we be?" In a bipolar emotional twist, she smiles. "But then I think of you, and a sense of happiness and hope lifts my spirit. Because I know you'll get well. You're one of the few on this ward I can say that to. You'll have plenty of time to make the world a better place by just being you."

That suggests I know who I am.

"Who are you, Madz?"

In the world of Shrinkdom, mind-reading should be considered cheating.

She sits across from me. "Madz?"

Pretty sure we've established I'm Madz, Harper. "I'll let you know when I figure that out." I hate therapy talk.

"You've spoken about sick kids you've seen these past few months, but you haven't said much about yourself. I know you were Madz the skater. An amazing skater from what I hear. You once described yourself as a cancer patient and said you didn't want anyone to know. You also mentioned you were adopted. Do any of those things influence who you are, Madz?"

Holy shit, she's literally in love with my name. "Hmm, let me think about that, Harper." Oh, yes, I did that. "I may have to get back to you on that one." I haven't spoken about my illness to people I've known for years. Why would I spill my guts to her?

The curability of my cancer doesn't make it suck any less, nor does it make it any easier to sit home and stew over who I am. "Maybe I can answer that question after I've had a chance to actually live outside the rink. Madz the skater? I knew who she was. Madz the regular bipedal hominid? Never spent much time with her. When I finally had the chance to, I got diagnosed with cancer."

"I get it. But just so you know, you're more than Madz the skater and Madz the girl with cancer. You can be both or neither, but inside those two girls is one person with, from what I've seen, a strong spirit and a good heart. You're so kind for taking on Chelsea's wish." She leans forward and furrows her brow. "Although at any point, you can pass the responsibility to someone else if you think this is too much for you. If it makes you too sad or if you're too tired or nauseous. I could figure out the logistics if I had to."

"I'll figure it out."

"I understand you're getting over an illness, and your own body's weak. But your nurse says you're on the upswing."

"Until the next round."

"Your final round." She smiles and nods. "That's huge. You have a curable type of cancer. You, Madz Monroe, will improve and have a happy and productive life." Her smile flattens out. "I know this is hard to hear, but regarding Chelsea . . ."

"We don't have much time."

She shakes her head. "Can we get you and her on the ice by the weekend?"

I text Nathan: *I realize you've gone above and beyond already, but I need at least a half hour of ice with no one else around.* I tell him about Chelsea's last wish and say: *Can you go on the ice with her and me? She needs someone to hold her up, and I'm not strong enough.*

He responds: *Sunday 8-9 a.m. Competition out of town this*

weekend—only a couple of skaters booked ice on the nine-o'clock session. I'll tell them the session's canceled. Will go on the ice with you.

I text him three hearts.

TWENTY-ONE

"**A**re you ready?" Mom asks.

"I think so," I say, following her to the car.

"I'm worried about your doing this. Do you feel up to it?"

"Barely, but not for physical reasons."

We get in the car, and she drives to the rink.

I "worked out" yesterday and early this morning to prepare for skating with Chelsea. Each time, I spent twenty minutes on my exercise bike, twenty seconds jumping rope, and twenty minutes stretching, the best I could do. After, I put on my skates (guards covering the blades) and went through the motions of a spin. I got dizzy. Same when I tried a flip jump. I'd hoped to do a few tricks for Chelsea, but she'll understand my limitations.

My biggest fears have to do with my little friend. I'm afraid I'll break down and cry, knowing this is the last time I'll see her. I'm afraid she'll break with one wrong move. I'm afraid she'll die in front of me.

Why is it that when you want time to go by slowly, minutes become seconds? SuperEdge is twenty minutes from my house. Yet we're here already, as if Mom transported us with a snap of her fingers. Chelsea and her mother wait out front; Chelsea in a wheelchair, wearing a helmet.

"Ugh, I forgot it," I say.

"What?"

"The gift I was going to give her. I told her I'd have a surprise for her."

"I think this is a pretty good surprise." Mom waves to them and parks. "I'll grab your bag. Go see Chelsea."

At the entrance, Chelsea says, "I was afraid to go in without you." She holds my hand, and I help her stand. "Make sure I don't fall. I'm really wobbly."

Holding her hand is the only thing standing between me and a panic attack. Going through the doors of SuperEdge, and going through them with such a responsibility? *We're here,* I tell myself, *and this is Chelsea's special day.*

I suck in a deep breath and blow out. No time to feel sorry for myself, sorry I took for granted walking through these doors as a healthy person. Sorry I didn't tell my parents sooner how tired and sore I was. Who knows, I could have caught my cancer in its first stage.

Mom hands me my skate bag. It holds two pairs of skates, mine and an old pair I wore in first grade. While she and Theresa sit at a table, Chelsea and I sit on the bleachers. I show her the smaller pair of skates. "These were mine when I was your age. I wouldn't let my mother give them away. If you want, you can keep them."

"No, thank you. I don't think I'll be skating much after

today." She holds one while I put the other on her. "They're pretty."

When her skates are on, I take out mine. I dig a Sharpie out of my bag. "Will you autograph my skate for me? You're my best friend, and I think you're a superstar. I want to always remember you and me here." I rest my skate on her lap, and she signs it.

Her mother stands. "Careful, Chelsea, don't cut yourself."

"How does she think you'll cut yourself with these puffy covers on the blades?" I say, squeezing one.

Chelsea giggles. "They're almost as big as the pillows on my bed."

Once my skates are on, I hold her hand and walk her onto the ice. Nathan had better show up soon. He didn't put out a walker to help me hold Chelsea up. She's sliding all over the place. Hunched over, holding her as her feet slip out from under her, my back aches.

I lose the strength to hold her up, so I sit her by the boards. Here, she does something worse than out-and-out cry. She frowns. The corners of her lips dive downward, her chin twitches, and her eyes fill up. A blink empties the two big pools.

I'm a failure. I sit with her, and we rest our backs against the boards.

"Everything's too wobbly," she says.

"I'm sorry. That stinks. And you know what? I hate being sick. I hate even more that you're sick. If I had a magic wand, I'd wave it over you and make you all better." I wave the imaginary wand.

"That's what Mama says." She hugs my arm and rests her head on it. "My butt's cold."

Nathan shows up out of nowhere and snowplows Chelsea's and my legs. "Get up, lazybones."

"I can't," Chelsea says.

Nathan picks her up and sits her on a stack of two milk crates zip-tied together. "Madz, do your thing." Lindsey and I used to have so much fun pushing each other around on this thing.

I hold on to the back of the crate, and Chelsea grips my wrists. "Hold on tight," I push gently at first, then harder. Chelsea screeches a happy screech I didn't think she had the energy for.

"This is fun," she says. She lets go of my wrists and holds out her arms. "Look, I'm flying."

I grip her waist with my left arm and push the crate with my right as we curve to our left. Then, I push her straight ahead, and Nathan skates backward in front of us, telling Chelsea, "Try to catch me." He lets out a ghoulish laugh. This is *not* the Nathan I've known for six years.

My neck, shoulders, and back ache. That and Mom's concerned facial contortions remind me I'm a different Madz from the one who used to race around this rink, thinking it wasn't big enough. Despite the aches, breathing this cool air soothes my insides.

"Doesn't that cold air feel good in your throat, Chelsea?" I ask.

"Yeah," she says. "Go faster." I manage to push her two more times around the rink. The whole time, in the back of my mind, I worry if she'll fall off and break her bones. She starts coughing, so Nathan carries her off the ice and puts her in the wheelchair. Theresa covers her and Buzzy, Chelsea's stuffed bee, with a blanket.

"Meet me at the table by the snack bar," Nathan says, running off.

"Here," Chelsea's mother says. She hands me my old, tiny skates.

I outgrew them, but Chelsea never will.

I pack up and meet the others at a table near the snack bar. Nathan brings us a tray of hot chocolates with whipped cream. He treats himself to a cup, a big deal because he claims to have given up sugar years ago. "I put a little cool water in them so they're not too hot." He holds up his cup. "Cheers."

I follow his lead, but Chelsea doesn't. Instead, her eyes roll to the back of her head, and her little body straightens out and tightens up, jaw clenched, hands in fists, left arm jerking. She turns purple. Nathan and I look at each other wide-eyed.

"Should we call an ambulance?" Mom asks.

"No, it'll be over soon," Theresa says, rubbing her daughter's head, telling her she loves her. "We're done with the hospital. Right, Chelsea?" She turns to me, Mom, and Nathan. "The hospice nurse is coming to our home this afternoon. She'll hook Chelsea up to medications that will make her comfortable and stop these seizures once and for all."

Hospice. Heaven's waiting room.

TWENTY-TWO

SuperEdge sucked the life out of me. In my cropped lycra skating pants and my *I'd rather be skating* T-shirt, I plop into bed and seesaw between sleep and semi-consciousness. Until I hear the doorbell ring.

I slip out of bed and creep into the hallway, to the top of the stairs.

"I'm sorry. She's sick," Gallagher says.

"Again?" Will says.

"Yes," Gallagher says.

"With all due respect, sir, you're insulting my intelligence. You could at least try to concoct a different excuse."

"You're right, lad. Come in. You, too, lass."

The lass must be Gracie.

In a move of sheer defiance, Gallagher takes matters into his own hands and goes against my no-visitors policy. "You can see her if you want, but you'll have to wear this mask and social distance times two."

That's what you think, buddy. Although, I would like to see Will's face when Gallagher hands him a mask with a funny graphic on it—a distorted smile, a mustache, or puckered lips. Gallagher bought a bunch of them. He's loosened up since getting a cell phone from this century, and I'm pretty sure he thinks he's a comedian.

"What's going on in here, some weird Munchausen's thing?" Will says. "This place smells like bleach. If you want Madz to get better, I suggest you open some windows."

Gallagher and Mom's doing. Bleach isn't my favorite scent, but it beats the smell of tuna and is definitely better than the smell of Dad and Gallagher's morning favorite, fried eggs. Yech. I turn, ready to race to my room and lock the door. I need to regroup from my morning with Chelsea before diving into a discussion about broken promises and dropping off the map for three months. Will speaks again, and I freeze.

"Gracie, forget about visiting the eternally sick patient with the never-ending doctor appointment." He texts me: *You shouldn't recruit your butler to do your dirty work. Being rich gives you no right to hurt my sister. If you want her out of your life, tell her. She can handle the truth better than you think.*

"Let's go, Gracie," he says.

"There," Gracie says, pointing up the staircase at me.

I duck behind a wall.

"I saw her!" she yelps, as if proclaiming a rare Sasquatch sighting. "You go check on Mom, Will. I'm visiting Madz."

She stomps up the stairs as I race to my room.

"No!" Will yells up the stairs. "Come with me, Gracie, right now. I mean it. If Madz wanted to see you, she would have come down by now."

"No!" She stops in my doorway and traps me in her gaze, sabotaging my plan to hide in my closet.

"Please don't go in her room, Gracie!" Mom hollers up the stairs.

Gracie's phone buzzes. She looks down at it, then back at me. "You really are sick." She's wearing the mask printed with full red lips in a giant smile showing off pure-white teeth.

"I'll be better soon." I sit in my bed and pull the covers over my legs.

She stares at me, looks at her phone, then stares at me again. No freaking out. Good. I take it she's not shocked by my appearance.

"I'm surprised Will drove you here. I figured he'd be too mad at me to let you see me."

"I forced him to. Anyway, I thought we were friends."

"We are."

"No." She shakes her head. "Friends don't lie to friends. A doctor appointment doesn't take three months. You said you'd help me with skating and Will with landscaping. Summer's almost over, and that's Will's busiest season. And you told Nathan you didn't want to come to the rink anymore because it was too hard. But you went to see Joao." She sits in the doorway, her crinkled brow throwing shade on the bright grin masking her. "You didn't even wave to me."

"I didn't tell Nathan that. He assumed it." Now I really am lying. "No. Here's the truth. Nathan said that because I gave him strict orders to keep my illness a secret."

"You have cancer. I can tell. You have no hair under your hat, and your face looks puffy. You don't look like yourself. Sorry, I don't mean to be rude."

"It's okay. You can be honest. This mirror here has been brutally truthful." I wave a hand toward it.

"If you really wanted me to be your friend, you would have told me." Elbows on her knees, she rests her chin on her two fists. "I could have helped you."

I close my eyes, hoping she'll magically disappear when I open them, so I won't have to work through this. I open them, and yup, she's still here. Will says Gracie can handle the truth. So I serve it hot on a platter the way she does. "Every person has to decide for herself how to deal with certain situations, Gracie. Don't judge me because I made a choice that fit me better than you."

She points her finger at me. "Rude." She shakes her head. Like the stress trenches on her forehead, her tone mismatches her cartoon smile. "If you told me you were sick, it wouldn't *fit* me"—she tugs her T-shirt—"like this. It wouldn't fit me to have to help you either. But I would do it because that's what friends do. They help each other like you were supposed to help me with my skating."

By not letting my condition affect her honest approach to matters, Gracie has not let me down. The girl is a well-oiled truth-telling machine. Lies are like clunkers. They require constant upkeep, and you never know when they'll break down. I'm done with them.

"I'm sorry I hurt you, and thank you for caring about me. You're a good person. But I *did* help you with skating. Do you have amnesia? And FYI, when I couldn't help you in person, I helped behind the scenes."

She plants her eyes on her phone.

Her response prompts me to calm my tone. "Sorry if that

was too harsh." She continues to stare at her phone. "I heard you passed your maneuvers test. Congratulations."

. . .

"*Hello*, Gracie."

"Thank you." She continues to stare at her phone.

Gallagher shows up, his cheeks glowing red bulbs. "Gracie, you need to go with Will now." He eyes me. "Madz, please come down."

"I can't."

"I think you should." He hands me a mask. Weird. It's a plain one—no silly print. Something's wrong.

Gracie sits in the doorway, stares at the floor, and pulls off her mask. "I don't need this if Madz is wearing one."

Gallagher extends his hand to Gracie. "Let's go see your brother, young lady." He didn't call her *lass*. He means business.

She slaps his hand away. "No."

"Young lady—"

"No." Gracie hugs her knees and rocks. "She always says she's going to kill herself. Will said I didn't have to go with him the next time she said it."

Mom group-texts Gallagher and me: *Gracie has to stay here. (Keep your distance, Madz.) I'm going with Will. Your father will be home soon.*

Gallagher and I look up from our phones. His brow wrinkles, mirroring mine. He nods toward Gracie.

I sit on the floor, about five feet away from her. The longest moment of silence in history passes. "I told you a secret, and it was a big one. I'm sick. You were right. I do have cancer. Did. The doctor thinks my chemotherapy got rid of it. But sometimes chemo makes me sick and tired too."

Eyes to the floor, she nods her head slowly.

"Now it's your turn, Gracie. Can you tell me the truth about why my mother had to leave with Will?" The reason must be drastic considering Mom referred to him as a "little shit" only a few months ago.

She raises her head slowly. "My mother has something worse than cancer. She has forever sadness." Her gaze drifts toward a window. "She cries all the time. When she argues with my father, she threatens to kill herself, but she never does. She just says it to get his attention."

Gallagher sits near Gracie, and now we're all on the floor because what else is there to do?

Above the cloud we're riding, sparkles dance on my chandelier. I loved how they danced on my crystal-embellished figure-skating dresses, too, under the spotlights of that world. It was a protective bubble shielding me from this dark place I've spiraled into, where kids battle cancer, parents kill themselves, and siblings are pushed into parenting roles. When I walked out of SuperEdge that hot day in May, little did I know I threw myself into the wolves, a pack called "Real Life." How does an expert skater, a pro at gliding through a specific, secluded world, pilot this one, a bottomless pit of despair?

The doorbell rings. Gracie runs into my room, looks out the window, runs into my closet, and shuts herself in.

"Jesus, Mary, and Joseph, and all the saints in Heaven, now I have to bleach the whole room down again," Gallagher says, getting on all fours, wincing as he stands. While he answers the door and Gracie hides in my closet, I rest my face in my hands, wondering what else is coming.

A few minutes later, Gallagher arrives at my bedroom door

with one Marsha Meriwether. She sports a blue disposable mask and wants to see how Gracie is "weathering the storm."

"Where is she?" Mrs. Meriwether asks.

I point to the door Gracie's behind.

The stranger enters my room and taps the closet door. "Gracie, would you mind coming out? Nothing bad will happen."

"Duh, something bad did happen, or you wouldn't be here."

"Can I open the door?"

Gallagher watches from the doorway, shaking his head, mirroring my dumbfounded headshake. Both of us have turned into bobbleheads. When Gracie opens the closet door, he disappears into the hall.

"You can't take me away, Marsha," Gracie says. "I won't live with strange people who might be freaks."

An ironic statement, given Gallagher's peeking into the room, wearing a mask with a mustache.

My room has never seen so much action, and it's wearing me out. I burrow deep under my comforter and pull it over my head.

"See what you did?" Gracie says to Marsha. "You made Madz have to lie down and hide. You're stressing her out, and she has cancer. You told me you help kids."

I hear her panting, so I peek from under my covers. She has that piercing look in her eyes. Uh-oh, it's coming. Blocking my ears, I imagine Marsha's reaction to Gracie's screaming. Then I smile and fight off highly inappropriate giggles. It's so refreshing to hear a young person bugle a healthy shrill.

TWENTY-THREE

The garage door hums open at midnight. Will texts me: *Thanks for watching Gracie. I'm sorry you've been so sick. (Your mother told me.) We should talk sometime.*

Shivering from the AC, I wrap myself in my pink fleece robe, put on my slippers, and head downstairs.

Mom washes her hands. "I can't hug you. I still have hospital germs on me. Is your father sleeping?"

"Yeah, on the couch in his office. He didn't want to go to bed until you came home."

"Sit down for a minute," she says, sitting at the table. "I told Will about you. About why you didn't want anyone to know. I hope you're not mad, but we were alone in the car, and he'd just learned of his mother's death. She overdosed. I also thought it was important for him to understand you hadn't abandoned him and his sister. I told him how you helped them and that it was the best you could do under the circumstances."

"I'm not mad you told him."

"He figured you influenced Nathan to help his sister. Will just couldn't get past your disappearance."

"Did his mother leave a note?"

"No, but she'd threatened this before and was hospitalized a couple of times as a result. Is Gracie asleep?"

"Sounded like she was. The girl's got a mean snore." Before leaving, Marsha Meriwether conference-called Mom, Will, and my father, who was in his office. (Gracie and I eavesdropped.) They agreed Gracie should stay at my house until things settle down at hers. "How is Will? I hope he's not alone in that house." I heard Marsha say Mr. Cruz is in rehab.

"Will is putting up a solid front. He won't sleep here. Too proud. That boy acts a lot older than his age. He reminds me of your father when I first met him." She sits at the table, burying her head in her hands. "That doesn't change the fact Will's too young to be going through this. I'm sorry I was so hard on him for giving you the money for your test."

Gallagher pops out of his room and says, "Will he be okay? What's going to happen with Gracie in the long run?" He fills the kettle with water. Stressful times call for tea, but so do all other times when you're him.

"Will says he won't let Gracie go into their father's custody, and the social worker is on Will's side. The father's in rehab. When he's sober, Mrs. Meriwether says she'll reassess the situation."

"I know where this is going." Mom acts tough, but a little-known fact about her is she hates to see anyone without a home or family. My birth mother and I were homeless while Mom served as my birth mother's public defender. Mom got us into public housing and continued to follow our case closely. She and Dad adopted me after the overdose.

And Gallagher? They sort of adopted him too. His wife died of a heart attack shortly after they immigrated here from Ireland to live with their son and daughter-in-law. Shortly after that, his son, daughter-in-law, and unborn grandson died. Mom knew the lawyer who prosecuted the drunk driver who killed them. She followed the proceedings and became friends with Gallagher, who, she claims, was a lost soul at the time. He'd been recently diagnosed with diabetes and had no family in the US other than the ones buried.

Mom represented Gallagher pro bono and got him a healthy settlement for his losses. She didn't settle his loneliness, though, until she offered him a place in her home. A package deal that included Dad and me. Some people need money; others need a family.

"Your father and I told the social worker that Will and Gracie could stay here until their father completes his treatment program," Mom says.

"You said Will won't sleep over," I say. "What will they do with him? He's not eighteen yet."

"His age is irrelevant. He's been emancipated for over a year. Most kids leave home after being released from their parents' custody. Will stayed to help his family."

"Wow, wow, wow." I slowly shake my head.

"You can say that again," Gallagher says, taking teabags out of a canister. "That lad had to grow up too fast. Such a pity."

Dad comes out of his office, yawning. "He turned out to be a responsible young man. A solid individual." He pecks Mom on her forehead and sits with us.

Images of Will project in my mind: working hard landscaping, speaking with Gracie, speaking for Gracie, taking my trash at UdderBuds Ice Creamery, asking me to honor my promise to his sister. He's been parenting her. Alone. At least my parents and Gallagher have cared for me during my extended crisis. Who cared for Will during his, before Mom showed up?

Mom looks at me. "What did Gracie do when Mrs. Meriwether showed up?"

"She's a tough cookie, that Gracie," Gallagher says. "Gave Mrs. Meriwether a piece of her mind, she did."

"She hid in the closet and screamed at the top of her lungs," I say. "But when Marsha said Gracie could sleep at our house, Gracie snapped out of her attitude and acted as if nothing unusual had happened."

"You call the case worker Marsha?"

I shrug. "Gracie does."

The kettle boils. "None for me, Gallagher, and decaf for the rest of you," Mom says.

"None for me, thanks," I say.

Mom gets up and rewashes her hands. "Madz, did you tell Gracie your room is off-limits for the time being? You can't get sick. We're so close to O and D." That's Mom lingo for *over and done with*.

"Oh, speaking of which," Mom continues, "I checked your patient portal, Madz." She serves Dad his tea. A small amount spills as her shaky hands place it on the table. "Your neutrophils are up, and the rest of your labs are good. You're going into your last treatment in good shape."

I sigh in relief. "I set the ground rules with Gracie. Personal space, germ consciousness—"

Mom gasps. "I haven't asked you how you're feeling. I know your labs are good, but how are you? So much has gone on between Chelsea and Gracie . . ."

The woman's jittery. She nibbles the skin around her

thumb, rewashes her hands, and grabs a bottle of water from the fridge.

"How much coffee did you drink?" Dad asks her.

"Three cups." She sits next to me. "Tell me, Madz. Any nausea? Fever?" She presses her palm against my head.

Dad once argued Mom should stick to decaf. He said she didn't need caffeine because she was already wired like a squirrel.

"I'm fine. Tell me about Will. How'd he take it? I mean, he just lost his mother."

"He went to his night job, stocking shelves at a grocery store." She shakes her head. "It's not right. I don't know when he sleeps. In a couple of months, he'll start a paid internship at a landscape architecture firm. He got that and a few thousand dollars for winning the landscaping competition this summer. You'd think he'd work less after receiving extra money. My guess is he took the night job to occupy his mind."

"The boy landscapes all day," Gallagher says, sitting with us. "How can he do an internship?"

"Gallagher's right," I say. "There are only twenty-four hours in a day." Even "solid individuals" have time constraints and breaking points.

"He starts the internship after his fall cleanups," Mom says, "during his slow season. That way, he won't lose his customers or money. He makes more landscaping than he will as an intern, so the timing makes sense."

"I hope we have a warm winter," I say. "Don't forget, he added snow-plowing to his winter-service menu, and he'll be in school."

"The internship will count as work-study hours, which will consolidate the school workload, but that boy has the weight of the world on his shoulders." Mom rests her head in her hands. "He pays the family's bills *and* parents Gracie. Doctor appointments, making sure the school follows her ed plan." She looks up at me. "Don't tell anyone. That's his personal business."

"You forgot to say he takes her skating and pays for it," I say. "Didn't his father work before going into rehab?" I cross my arms on the table and rest my head on them, struggling to keep my eyes open.

"The father's allegedly an alcoholic and a gambler. He allegedly gambled and drank away his paycheck every week."

I pop my head up. "You're talking to your family, Mom. You don't have to say *allegedly*."

"He's been in rehab for a week," Mom says. "Will thinks his mother overdosed because she'd thought her husband left the family for good. Will couldn't convince her otherwise." She finishes her glass of water and kisses my forehead. "Get to bed. We need you rested and strong for your final treatment Friday."

"We can't have this drama affecting your health," Dad says. "C'mon. Your mother and I will walk you to your room." He dumps what's left of his tea in the sink.

"Drama?" Sounds distant and cold, so . . . motion-picturey. "We're talking about Will and Gracie's lives, Dad, and their parents' lives. This affects my feelings, not my health. I care about what's going on with them." Those words flick on a switch in my brain, helping me understand why Gracie and Will would be upset about being left in the dark about my condition.

I stand up. "Wait. Did Will and Gracie's father leave rehab to go to the hospital? Does he know what happened?"

"Good question, Madz," Gallagher says, sipping his tea.

"Yeah, good question," Dad says, running his fingers through his silver crown. He yawns.

"Yes, he knows, and no, he didn't leave rehab," Mom says. She shakes her head. "I can't understand how a father couldn't take a few hours to be with his son under these circumstances."

"Maybe he was afraid of going off the wagon if he left the rehab," I say.

"I can't imagine Will and Gracie having no extended family to take them in," Dad says.

"I can imagine it," Gallagher says.

Mom rests her hand on his shoulder.

Everything she told me sinks in. "I joked with Will once about how he acted like he was Gracie's father. He said he may as well be." I've officially solved the may-as-well-be mystery. I may have hidden my illness from him, but he hid a condition of his own. I can't blame him for responding to Lindsey's flirtation or dating Heels. He deserves to feel special. He deserves a break from the nightmare he's been living.

"Will's been a father to his parents too," Mom says. "But to your point, Mason, one family member is trying to help: Will and Gracie's great-aunt, the younger sister of their paternal grandfather. She told Mrs. Meriwether she'd fly up from Florida to help Will with Gracie while their father's in rehab. If necessary, she'll take Gracie home to Florida with her. She's arriving tomorrow afternoon."

"I'll make them a nice dinner tomorrow," Gallagher says, bringing his mug to the sink. "I'll take it to Will's house to keep Madzy safe. Yes, that's what I'll do." He sits at his little desk in the kitchen and grabs a pencil and a piece of paper, his usual meal-planning procedure.

"We'll do it here," Mom says. "Gracie should eat with her

family, and it's too soon for her to see where her mother passed. Madz's counts are good enough." She hugs Gallagher. "You're so sweet."

"Aw, aren't you sweet?" Dad says, hugging Gallagher.

"All right, that's enough," Gallagher says.

"Dad, this isn't a joke." I gently whack his arm. "Something terrible happened. Is happening."

"What happened, happened. We can still be happy. Life goes on," he says.

"C'mon, Madz," Mom says. "Get to bed. You, too, Gallagher." She holds Dad's arm. "We're all sleep-deprived."

Mom and Dad walk me to my room. Dad follows me in. Still in the clothes she wore at the hospital, Mom watches from the door. I slip under the covers, and Dad tucks me in for some reason. Then he joins Mom in the doorway.

"Thanks for going to the hospital with Will, Mom. I know you won't sleep because of it. You didn't have a glass of wine to calm you down."

"You know what helps me sleep at night?"

"What?"

"Knowing your dad and I raised a daughter who's a good person." She blows me a kiss. I pretend to catch it and place it on my cheek, like she used to do when I was little and blew her a kiss from the rink.

I wish what she said was true, but I'm not a good person. "I was mean to you when I left skating, and I was mean to you when you cried when we found out I had cancer. I was a sucky person for doing that. Sorry."

"You have nothing to be sorry about." They shut my door, and I peek at my phone. Joao texted me a smiley face. Nathan texted me: *Thinking of you* [*heart emoji*]. Both messages are from four in the afternoon, the start of Joao's lesson, and they're perfectly enough. I text Joao a smiley face and Nathan a *Thank you:)*

My heartbeat kicks into overdrive when I think about texting Will, but I won't get a wink of sleep if I don't text him. What do I say? "I'm sorry about your mother"? He doesn't deserve generic condolences. Nor does he need a reminder about his mother while he's working, trying to distract himself from the harsh reality of her death.

I text: *Thank you for trusting us with your sister. I hope I see you soon [heart].*

MY ROOM IS TOO DARK, and it's frigid. Someone set the AC too low. I burrow deeper under my covers, pulling them up to my ears, and check the time on my phone: 3:30 a.m.

Tingles creep up my spine, and I have a strong feeling I'm not alone, that someone who's not among the living is watching me.

I've sensed this before. Mom says it happens when a person's partially asleep. Lindsey blames the "bewitching hour." Between three and four o'clock in the morning, spirits visit because darkness and fatigue lower a person's guard and open a spiritual portal.

Normally, when I wake at the bewitching hour, I cover my head, frozen out of legit fear, and Our Father and Hail Mary myself back to sleep. But this time, I'm not scared. My guest can't be Will's mother; I never met her. Even if I did, I would expect her spirit to beeline it to her daughter's room and not make a pit stop in mine.

The energy wraps around me, warm and comfortable. I'm sensing *Hi, friend.* My skin prickles and breaks out with goosebumps. They ride up the back of my neck and on my head. . . . *My head.*

"Hi, friend," I say. A second round of goosebumps rise and fall, and I go from content to devastated. I know who it is. I close my eyes, and a memory reels of Chelsea, her studying the wings of the blue butterfly as if mentally creating a pattern of their design.

Groggy, I Our Father and Hail Mary my way into a dream . . .

I'm skating, stroking the ice hard and fast. I mohawk into back crossovers and push hard. I step forward onto my left outside edge, thrust my right knee up, pull into a tight spin in the air, and check out as my toe pick smacks down on the ice for a solid landing. Clean double axel. Like I used to do before my strength packed up and left me.

I'm doing a triple next, I think, knowing I can and wanting to feel the rush of flight. Stroking hard and fast, I speed around the ice. The cool air blows through my hair, my lungs drink up the breeze, and I wish there were a marathon for skaters, twenty-six miles of ice. And I'm happy, even when I wake up before pulling off the triple.

TWENTY-FOUR

Today, Monday, I learned three things: (1) A basic cremation costs \$1395.00, including transportation of the deceased, copies of the death certificate, and, among other things, the container the ashes go into. (2) I could be a psychic medium because (3) Chelsea passed away.

I learned number one when Will came over after work, before he picked up his aunt from the airport. Mom had insisted upon looking at his cremation contract. (She also insisted he and his aunt eat dinner at our house tonight.) I learned numbers two and three after Theresa texted Mom this morning.

Her eyes jumped from her phone to me.

"Chelsea," I said.

Mom nodded.

I walked to the backyard and sat behind the poolhouse, next to a bed of dandelions. I pulled a couple but soon surrendered. "You won," I said, tossing the picked weeds. Leaning back against the poolhouse, I took out my phone and searched a weird phenomenon Mom once told me about: *death comes in threes.*

The search turned into a rabbit hole of bad things to do with the number three. A search suggestion, *when will I die*, turned up at the bottom of the first page. One search led to another, and I eventually stumbled upon a live "world deaths" clock. It's similar to the running US Debt Clock but counts mortality instead of dollars. And guess what? People are dropping like flies, unlike the national debt, which keeps rising.

Safe to say that on a world scale, people die in much larger clumps than threes. This was enough to discourage me from entering what would have been my next search: *cancer deaths per year.*

Why bother? Plenty of other things kill people. If cancer doesn't do it, something else will. I could be cured of cancer and then die in a freak accident like Gallagher's son and daughter-in-law. Everything is borrowed in this life. Time, the soft light of sunrise and sunset, the bright light of midday, the joy you get from a smile, and the big one: life itself. We're all Cinderella, dancing, swirling around, ignoring the clock while time zooms in on our stroke of midnight.

Pasta, a roast, potatoes, string beans, and salad sit on the kitchen table. On the counter sits a box of pastry Mom picked up from the bakery. Two untimely deaths within twelve hours, and we're hosting a feast. I guess that's one way to deal with death. If you can't beat it, eat.

And Will eats. His eyes fix on his plate and stay there, even as his Aunt Elaine asks him questions about school, work, and Gracie. He responds with one-word answers, mainly "Okay" and "Yup." Kind of uncomfortable to witness. After all, his aunt's an older woman, and she flew up from Florida out of concern for him and his sister.

"Elaine," Mom says, "did you know Will won a landscape-design contest? One of the awards was an internship at an architectural design firm in Boston."

Will has gone from eating to moving food around with his fork.

"Good for you, Will," Aunt Elaine says. "Your mother once told me how much you loved helping her plant flowers when you lived on Maple Street."

Will puts his fork down and wipes his mouth. "It was a very happy time in our lives. Too bad my father gambled the house away, huh?" Looking at his plate, he sighs. He looks up at her. "Sorry." He glances at my parents and me. "Sorry."

My hand twitches, itching to reach across the table for his but reluctant. His hand slides closer to mine but falls short of touching my skin. Mom seated me at the end of the table, an empty chair on either side of me. My counts are better, but we're still being careful. However, fear of physical contact isn't why I'm reluctant to extend my hand another inch and grip his fingers.

How can it be that we've been through so much together without actually being together? By now, holding hands should be second nature to us. Cancer and suicide have invaded our relationship like poison ivy, forcing us into emotional hazmat suits.

Aunt Elaine shakes her head. "That was a terrible thing your father did, Will. I'm sorry it happened. At least he's trying to get help now. That's a big step for him."

No wonder Will okayed and yupped his way through their conversation earlier. He shouldn't have to discuss this in front of all of us. Before his mother died, he dealt with hardship in his own way on his own terms. Without the help or hassle of anyone else's two cents.

He catches me staring at him. Our eyes speak to each other for a few seconds. His tell me he's angry and vulnerable but as strong as a stone cliff as he takes a beating from these crashing waves of memories and emotions. My eyes try to convey, *Let's talk in private as soon as we have a chance.* Despite the stone facade, he's still human.

"Will didn't want to move from that house," Gracie says. "He cried when my mother said we had to leave. He didn't want to leave the garden they made. Right, Will? We had to leave your garden there."

If I could drag Will away from this table, where his most personal laundry is being aired, I would. Clearly, he's not the open book Gracie is. He and I shift in our seats.

"Excuse me." Will stands. "Thank you, Mr. and Mrs. Monroe. This was really nice of you. I have to get to my night job." He looks at me and cracks a smile. "Bye." He taps his sister's shoulder. "Be good, Gracie. I'll see you tomorrow." He leaves.

"Awkward," Gracie says as Will walks out the door.

"More like bad manners," Aunt Elaine says. "I know he's been through a lot, but that's no excuse for being rude."

I open my mouth in a silent gasp. Mom and I have a meeting of the eyes before she shifts her attention to Aunt Elaine.

"He really does have to go to work," Mom tells her. "And he's been anything but rude since I've known him." She clears Will's plate off the table and joins Gallagher at the sink.

Mom has officially redeemed herself from the fiasco she put

me through after finding out Will loaned me money. I bolt from the table and stand on the front porch as Will approaches his truck. "Will." He turns to me, too far away for a hug, too rushed for a meaningful conversation, too special for a cliché. "Talk to you later, okay?"

He nods and waves before taking off.

I should have run to the truck and hugged him to make up for my inability to form a proper sentence. One that would express my admiration for him, how much I care about him, and how unfair I think his situation is.

I return to the kitchen table and sit. So does Mom.

"Will isn't rude. He's just mad," Gracie says to her aunt. "He thinks if you really cared"—she forks a potato—"you would have checked on us when my mother was in the hospital while my father was on vacation for a month." She pops the potato into her mouth.

"I'm sorry, Gracie. I had no idea your father took off for that long," Aunt Elaine says.

Gracie shakes her head, swallows her potato, and points at her target. "That's a fib, Aunt Elaine. Marsha told me she asked if you heard from him. She said I might have to go to your house. Will told her he'd watch me, then Mum came home cuz she felt better. That's why Marsha didn't make me go with you."

Aunt Elaine tilts her head, the "eleven" between her brows deepening. "Was that in October of last year?"

"Yes. Me and Will put up Halloween decorations, and Mum ripped them down right before we called 911 to take her to the hospital."

"I do remember." She looks at my parents. "You have to understand. My husband was in hospice at that time, dying of leukemia. I couldn't deal with a dying husband and Gracie's mother's calls. She'd be frantic, and I'd have to calm her down. I'd already tried for years to convince my nephew, Gracie's father, to get help. I asked Mrs. Meriwether if there were any signs of, you know"—she hand-shields her lips from Gracie's view and mouths the word *abuse*—"and she said no."

I think most people would agree that a father gambling away the family home and a mother ripping down her children's decorations qualify, on some level, as abuse.

Aunt Elaine turns to Gracie. "Uncle Pete's in Heaven now. I have plenty of time to give you my full attention. If your father says it's okay, you can live with me."

Gracie crosses her arms. "That's so funny I forgot to laugh. Papa doesn't say okay to where I live; Will does. Besides, I don't need to live with you. I'm living with Madz until I can go home with Will. I don't even know you. You're a stranger."

Aunt Elaine rolls her eyes. "Will is always working, and I'm not a stranger. Your grandfather was my older brother."

"I'm Will's helper. And I'm old enough to stay home when he's at his night job. I'm not stupid. I'll just go in my room and lock the door when Papa gets home, so he won't yell at me."

"Well, Gracie, I don't think it's right that you should have to lock yourself in your room. You wouldn't have to do that at my house."

"Stranger danger!" Gracie yells, pointing at her aunt. Shifting gears, my fiesty friend drops her pointer, turns to me, and calmly says, "Madz, can we watch a movie now?"

Mom gives me a nod, signaling me to grant Gracie's wish.

I, of all people, get why Aunt Elaine's husband's illness stole her attention from Gracie and Will's plight. The geographical distance worsened the detachment. But being their aunt should have meant something to her. Why would she maintain "stranger" status knowing what her two minor relatives were going through? I'm starting to see Gracie's honesty as an invaluable survival tactic. She, no doubt, picked up that trait from Will.

"Nice meeting you," I say.

In the movie room, Gracie pulls a pack of sour gummy rolls from the display cabinet, reclines in her chair, and bites off a piece of the candy strip. I sit two seats away from her.

"I won't live with a strange old lady," she says. "When I can't stay here anymore, I'll go back home with Will. I'm not a baby. I'm going to be fifteen in three months." She adjusts her seat back to its original position and stands.

"Where are you going?"

"Spying."

I follow her out of the room, down the hall, to the staircase. She squats behind the potted parlor palm, a tigress peering through the leaves, stalking her aunt. I pray the adults don't say anything that could freak Gracie out. Tempted to clear my throat to give them the heads-up, I hold back so Gracie doesn't think I'm trying to sabotage her.

I throw germ-caution to the wind and crouch behind the plant with her. "Move over," I whisper.

While Gallagher and Dad clear the table, Mom says to Elaine, "I think you need to discuss Gracie with Will. He's her primary caretaker."

"He's so young, though."

"Yes, he is, Elaine, but from what he told me, he's been running the household since he was fifteen. You can't just take his sister down to Florida without discussing it with him. He has rights. He'll soon be eighteen, and more important, he's been emancipated since he was sixteen. He has proven he's responsible."

Mom's learned a lot about Will since his mother died, but I'm sure she's also done her research. She'd never advocate for him without confirming anything he told her.

"My whole life is in Florida—my friends, my home. I want to help, but I can't stay in Massachusetts indefinitely. We have great programs in my community for kids like Gracie. She won't want for anything."

Gracie's chest rises and falls in giant waves, each ferocious breath gusting through her clenched teeth with a "shh." I tap her arm and signal a shush. Miracle of miracles, her breathing settles.

"I hear what you're saying," Mom says, "but do you know Gracie loves to skate? And from what I hear, she does a good job helping Will with his landscaping work. She has a good routine here and has thrived despite her parental situation."

"She can get into a good routine in Florida. When my nephew gets out of rehab, Mrs. Meriwether could let Gracie live with him. What happens if he goes back to drinking and gambling? Is Gracie supposed to lock herself in her room every night while Will's working? Unless that boy can get his own apartment—"

"That *is* his apartment. Who do you think has been paying the rent? Look, this isn't my decision to make. Legally, it's Gracie's father's. If he gets his act together. Realistically, Will should have the final say. In fact, I'll represent him pro bono if anyone goes against what he thinks is best for his sister."

Gracie makes a tight fist and throws her thumb up.

Aunt Elaine sighs. "You're right. I just feel . . . so bad for him, you know? He's seventeen, and all he knows is work.

Whether it's tending to his business or caring for his sister or a sick parent. He needs a life. I feel terrible I didn't step in sooner. I was so upset at my nephew that I'd say things I shouldn't, and then he'd tell me to mind my own business. I'm the one who called CPS in the first place. Five years ago. I told them if the situation got to the point where the kids' safety was in jeopardy, I'd take them."

"Believe me, I've handled many cases involving children who should have been in a better environment. Your stepping in sooner probably wouldn't have made a difference. As long as protective-service authorities felt the kids were safe, they probably would've kept them in their home. Do you mind if I make a suggestion?"

"Of course not."

"Just be there for Will and Gracie. Ask Will what he thinks. Ask him what you can do to help. See where the conversation goes from there."

Elaine's visit comes to a close. As Mom walks her to the door, Gracie lies on the floor and clutches her chest. If she weren't so young, I'd think she was having a heart attack. She squeezes her eyes, milking tears, and her chest quakes. In an uncharacteristically quiet voice, she says, "My mother really killed herself, didn't she?" She opens her eyes, sniffles, and stares at me. "She's gone forever, isn't she? Say it. She's gone forever."

Yes, she's gone forever, just like my birth mother, Chelsea, and so many other people at any given minute. I lie next to her, my legs numb from crouching, and rest my hand on her chest-clutching hands. "I'm sorry, Gracie, but yeah."

Wincing as if in physical pain, she weeps in whispers. I keep my hand on hers. "It hurts; I know. But you have friends and family who are still here for you. Everything will be alright." I break down and cry myself, sad for Gracie, sad for Chelsea, and sad for four-year-old me, who tried to wake up her dead mother.

Footsteps move closer to the parlor palm. When they stop, I look up and see Mom and Dad peering down at Gracie and me. I barely remember my birth mother, but I know them. I wouldn't change one single quirk of theirs for anything in the world. All those years I skated, every minute I've spent in this house, they were protecting me from the kind of pain engulfing Gracie now. The kind of pain that would have plagued me after my birth mother's death had my parents not filled the void.

PART 3
"HEALING"

TWENTY-FIVE

I sit in my closet with the door shut, hoping to keep prying ears from hearing my tele-shrink call. The morning sun streams through the room's only window as Harper greets me. She says she's glad I took the initiative to contact her, that doing so "signals progress."

Progress in what? I want to ask. I'm freaked out. I know I'm freaked out. I don't want to be freaked out. Therefore, I face-called a person trained to de-freakify people.

"How are you, Madz?"

Here we go again. I'm already sick of hearing my name. "I'm not good. Not good at all."

"You're not good at all?"

If that's therapeutic bait, she'd better restock the chum bucket because I'm not biting. Inspire me, Harper. "No, I'm not."

"Hmm. You're approaching your final treatment, and your

medical reports look good. That's wonderful news. But"—she winces—"I heard little Chelsea passed away. I'm sorry, Madz."

. . .

"It's okay to cry."

Good, because that's what I'm doing, with or without your permission.

After an awkward minute of Harper being an active listener to my crying, I get the words out: "Too many bad things are happening all at once."

Her stress-lined expression mirrors mine, and so do her words: "Bad things are happening all at once?"

"Please, don't mirror me. Do. Not. Mirror. Me. Talk like a person, not a parrot."

"You sound angry, Madz."

Duh. "Of course I'm angry. A six-year-old girl just died, and she was basically the only friend I had during my cancer treatments. The one person I could talk to. You know . . . like a teammate. Two other kids I care about, fourteen and seventeen, they're suffering. Their mother just killed herself. I try to help and say the right things, but who can steer that ship? My life's a mess. If only I stayed in my skating program."

"That wouldn't have changed what happened to Chelsea or your friends' mother. And it wouldn't have changed what happened to you, Madz."

I. Know. My. Fricking. Name. I *will* tell her that if she doesn't watch herself.

"You're nearing adulthood. You're supposed to be laughing with friends, dating, and planning your future. Instead, you're dealing with sickness, sadness, and death—a tornado of circumstances that have left you in a 'mess,' as you call it. But is it such a mess? For example, you granted Chelsea a wish at the end of her life. In doing so, you helped her family too."

. . .

"When Chelsea had a seizure at the rink, she scared me. At the same time, the way her mother stroked her head, telling her they weren't going back to the hospital . . . I don't know. There was a sense of peace, like Chelsea was next in line on the runway, ready to take off to a better place. Chelsea had her mother.

"Gracie, the fourteen-year-old I know, her mother died by suicide. She overdosed. When Gracie absorbed that reality last night, her face contorted into the mask of tragedy, and she clutched her chest as if someone had torn her heart out. Her mother, who inflicted the pain, obviously wasn't there to comfort her. She'd abandoned her daughter."

"Hmm. When you say Gracie's mother abandoned her, I get the impression you think her mother should have thought beyond her depression. It makes sense you'd expect a mother to put her children before her own feelings, Madz. Unfortunately, when a person is so depressed they're suicidal, their mind has already spiraled into a dark hole. Gracie's mother, at that point, wasn't able to think of how her death would impact her children, at least not in a rational way."

I twist my wig hair as I used to twist my own hair during the thinking process. "I'll try to understand your take on this, but I still think it's very selfish of a mother to kill herself, especially when she has a daughter with special needs and a son who's been breaking his back to keep a roof over the family's heads."

"You know, Madz, when I hear your concern for Gracie and her brother and reflect on how you were a support system for little Chelsea, I'm impressed by your ability to advocate for others while going through your cancer journey."

I hate the word *journey*. It's so overused. "I'm not a cliché."

"What do you mean by that?"

"I'm not on a cancer *journey*. I don't blog about what I'm going through, and I don't find it adventurous to embrace my baldness. I hate being bald, I hate my chemo treatments, and I hate being dependent on people.

"Everything has been arranged for me my entire life. My parents arranged my training, schooling, and friendships, except my friendships with Will and Gracie. Even who my parents would be was arranged. Just when I'd decided to forge my own path, cancer hurled me into a riptide of dependency. Treatments, appointments, meals—all arranged. What have I completed that I started on my own?"

"Getting through cancer treatments is no small thing."

"Take that, for instance. After Friday, based on everything I've heard about my odds of being cured, I'll be considered a survivor. All because my mother took me to treatments my doctor prescribed, which my nurse, Candy, gave me because researchers discovered these medications after years of studying them. I didn't make any of it happen. Will and Gracie are the real survivors. Anything good in their lives, they made happen. Yet despite their ability to survive, they're struggling and suffering."

They didn't deserve to be kept in the dark about my illness, given the impression another person had abandoned them. If I'd opened up to Will, maybe he'd have opened up to me, and this unsung hero who supports his family might have felt he had some support too. I cheated him out of that, cheated a boy who has suffered the loss of his home, his garden, and his mother.

"I've always had whatever I wanted."

"Have you, Madz?"

"Look at my life." I aim my phone at a wall of clothes and shoes the morning sun glows on. "What do you think?"

"The question is, what do you think?"

Now she's playing hardball. I knew all her sweet talk in the past was an act. "Well, Harper, yes. I think I have gotten everything I've ever wanted." I know where she's going with this. "I mean, I have one tiny memory of my birth mother. I was hungry, so I walked into her room and tried to wake her up. I yelled at her to wake up, but she wouldn't.

"Other memories come in flashes—the police coming in; a man picking me up, telling me, 'Don't worry. Everything's okay'; a lady holding my hand, introducing me to my adoptive parents. I can't remember what I had or didn't have other than a mother who didn't wake up. I was too young. Consequently, as far as I can remember, I've always had whatever I wanted."

"Except that day, when you wanted your mother to wake up."

No one can tell me Harper doesn't have an evil streak in her.

"What about what you didn't want, Madz? Tell me about what you didn't want."

I didn't want you saying my name five thousand times. "I didn't want cancer." Does she think I have to dig deep for that one? I need a professional, lady.

She nods. The woman is getting paid for nodding. She has shut off verbal communication.

"I didn't want anyone to know I had cancer," I say to

Harper McNodder, my new name for her. "I didn't want to watch Gracie cry over her mother. I didn't want to feel her . . ."

"Pain? Because maybe you felt something similar before but pushed it so far back you'd forgotten?"

"Touché." I was waiting for a reference to my subconscious. "Since we're in the trenches of my psyche, I'll give you one more. I didn't want to know a child who died of cancer. Had I not met Chelsea, I wouldn't have to experience such painful sadness and guilt for saying this: I don't want to go to her wake. Or her funeral. I'm too afraid."

"Afraid of . . ."

Jeez, lady. "I don't know. I figured you'd diagnose this mysterious fear and give me some tools to deal with it."

"Hmm. Let's think about this. You told me before you're afraid of germs and people feeling sorry for you. If I recall correctly, you also told me you were afraid of people thinking you would die."

Congratulations, you can read your notes.

"Are you afraid those things will happen at the funeral?"

"No."

"I've seen videos of you skating, Madz. In them, you appear healthy and strong. Powerful. You know how to fly across the skating rink, in full control of what you're doing. You said your parents arranged your training, but you were alone out there on the ice. You did that. Then you got weaker because of mono and cancer."

"That about sums it up." Thanks for nothing. "I learned how to fly across the ice, not how to deal with death and profound sadness."

"My point is this: we know why you got weak, and we're fixing it. You're still the same Madz who flew across the rink.

Who fought for those jumps and spins. Who fought your most recent fears about having cancer. Yet, you say you're afraid to go to Chelsea's funeral.

"I'm curious, Madz. We've talked about a number of things. What in particular prompted you to call my office today of all days? I'm glad you did; I'm just curious."

I sigh, twisting my wig hair, pausing to consider the answer. "Cancer made me unable to see people without seeing germs attached to them. Cancer made me unable to see children playing and laughing without seeing them suffering and dying. And now, I can't imagine being capable of moving on and planning my life after seeing Chelsea lying in a casket, dead. Shouldn't I be in that casket? I'm older than she was. It's not fair Chelsea suffered her whole life."

Tears begin to flow. "It's"—hiccup—"just"—hiccup—"not fair. And it's not fair that Gracie and Will got screwed in the parent department. The whole world's suffering, and I had the nerve to be upset about my coach and parents pushing me."

"I'm hearing a couple of things, Madz. I'm hearing concerns consistent with survivor's guilt, a normal, understandable emotion for what you've been through. Everyone's cancer is different. Yours happens to be more curable than Chelsea's. It's a reality we can't change. I'm also hearing you're a bit overwhelmed by other people's suffering, which tells me you're an empathetic person. The key to being empathetic is learning how to not let it overwhelm you. But first, we need to find out *why* everyone else's suffering is overwhelming you, why you're so in tune with their pain. Could it be you're suffering yourself and haven't totally acknowledged it yet?"

One thing I learned from competing: if I felt sorry for myself when I fell, I'd never finish the program. What's so bad about not completing it? People would pity me, possibly think, *Poor Madz, she tries so hard, doesn't she?* Talk about a will-breaker. Thinking about those repercussions makes me regret my dramatic exit from SuperEdge and reminds me I must finish this current "program," my confrontation with Chelsea's death. It ties into concerns related to Will and Gracie.

"I don't want to see Chelsea dead. I can hardly breathe when I think of it. My heart races. What can I possibly say to comfort her parents? When Gracie grimaced through level-ten emotional pain last night, I was mad at myself for not knowing how to comfort her. And I don't know what to say to her brother.

"I have no idea what I'm doing, Harper. I need tools. That's why I called you today. Tell me what I have to do, and I'll do it. Because right now, I don't want to leave my closet."

"Madz, you're experiencing anxiety for a valid and understandable reason. You're dealing with heavy situations most teens don't have to deal with. Rather than think of the big, overwhelming picture, break it down. Chelsea. You're afraid to see her. You're anxious about it because your brain senses a threat. What's the threat? Can the shell of Chelsea, the body she left behind, hurt you? Can anything or anyone at the funeral hurt you?"

"No?"

"You knew her. You cared about her. She adored you, and her parents adore you. They told me as much. You're safe with them."

She also tells me I'll be safe with Mom, who, I told Harper, is going with me. This convinces me there's no threat, hence no reason to be fearful. As far as Gracie goes, Harper encourages me to ask myself the same question: *what about that situation threatens me?*

"Maybe some of that fear is what you've held inside since you were a tiny child and lost your own mother," Harper says. "That same child is you, now trying to support Gracie and Will through the loss of their mother. I'll do my part and ensure the social worker sets up psychological help for Gracie and her brother. Other than that, just be you. Gracie wants to stay with you because she appreciates you just the way you are.

"But, Madz, there's no magic 'tool' to make these uncomfortable situations comfortable. And as you feel better and your body heals, you'll start exploring the world outside the hospital and your home, and you'll begin to see again that there's more to life than sickness and sadness."

Her saying that reminds me of the day I worked with Will and Gracie. It was a good day, and they seemed happy despite what was going on in their home. Gracie has a brother who advocates for her and guides her like a parent. With the help of Nathan, she'll also have ice theater to distract her from the pain she's experiencing.

My parents were distraction magicians. They kept my eyes off life's harsh realities with their "smoke and mirrors": Super-Edge, my busy schedule, and my idyllic home. I had some nerve worrying about people pitying me. In truth, I pitied myself. When I told Mom to keep my diagnosis secret so people wouldn't forecast my death, I was the one who was afraid I'd die.

The faucets in my eyes fire up again. Worsening matters, I'm more aware than most that just because I can get over this type of cancer doesn't mean I can't get another type and end up like Chelsea. Death, death, death. I have to believe Harper's right—as I heal, I'll feel better and start living. I'll see more life in life. "Thank you," squeaks out of my throat. Time's up. Harper has another patient waiting for her.

"Do you have any friends from skating you trust enough to talk to or hang out with?" she asks.

"As I told you before, the person I thought was my best friend, the one I hung out with before I got cancer, hasn't called or texted me. As for the others, I didn't set the best example by walking off the ice. It's possible their parents don't want them associating with me."

"Before we hang up, Madz, I'm curious. You said your coach mentally prepared you for competing. What would he tell you right before you went on the ice to compete?"

"Focus, nail the required elements, and remember to breathe. You can do this. Have fun."

"I don't expect you to have fun at Chelsea's funeral, but I think the rest is good advice. Good luck, Madz."

TWENTY-SIX

Three days of broken sleep have primed me for Chelsea's funeral today, Thursday. She'll go straight to the grave; her parents decided against a wake. Although this relieved my fear of seeing her dead, the rush to get her into the ground appalls me.

"Don't judge," Mom says. "Chelsea's gone now, and her parents spent every second with her while she was alive."

On the way to the funeral, one foot out the door, Mom gets called into work. The lawyer covering for her got sick, and the trial's today. No one knows more about the case than Mom and that woman. Mom, who reassured Dad he shouldn't cancel his important meeting, so he called Chelsea's parents, gave them his condolences, and left.

"I'll drive myself," I say half-heartedly.

"No," Mom snaps. "Not after what happened two weeks ago. Wait until you're back to normal."

I'm relieved she said no, but that doesn't solve the problem.

"Ride service," I say, pulling up a ride app on my phone. My finger hovers over the *confirm* button. I can't tap it. The reason goes beyond my aversion to going into a potentially germy car with a potentially germy driver, a stranger. I can't go to the funeral alone. I want to go with someone I feel safe with. Someone who knows I'm frail, who could fortify me.

"I'd rather someone go with you," Mom says.

"Gallagher," Gracie says.

"He went to Boston for his yearly physical," I say.

Mom hugs me. "I am so sorry, but I have to be in court in an hour." She holds my shoulders and makes direct eye contact. "Listen. Chelsea's parents will understand if you can't make it. I know they will. Text Theresa a thoughtful message, or snail mail a sympathy card with a personal note." She lets go. "C'mon, Gracie, let's get you to camp. Do you have your lunch bag?"

Gracie holds it up. The camp is an activity-filled orientation to the high school she'll attend soon. On her way out, she tells me, "Call Will. He'll take you." She nods at Mom, saying, "He will."

"He has to work," I say.

"He's the boss," Gracie says. "He can take a couple of hours off." She shuts the door, leaving me alone in my house. I can't miss this funeral. I need to show Chelsea's parents I haven't forgotten them or their daughter. After avoiding Will for months, after witnessing what he's gone through, asking him to help me takes nerve. But I have a lot of them, and I have to get going.

Granted, nothing's more lame or humiliating than asking a guy who just lost his mother to take me to a funeral. However, peculiar circumstances have become a given in both of our lives. And if he comes, we'll have a chance to speak privately.

How will I begin the conversation?

I'll say one true thing, Hemingway's advice for curing writer's block and Gracie's sure-fire way to get her points across. I ask my phone to call Will.

He picks up after one ring. "Hey."

"Hey. I know you have to work. I didn't want to bother you." Two true statements. So far, so good.

"I'm getting ready for work. I need to make the most of the good weather and my most profitable season."

"I hate to interfere with your work plans. I wouldn't ask if I weren't desperate." Two more true statements. This is what you call being on a roll.

"Wouldn't ask what?"

"Uhm." I chew my lip. "Gracie said you might—I mean, you could, possibly. I mean . . ." This is what you call a fudging disaster.

"What's up, Madz? Just say it."

Here we go. "Will you take me to a funeral? Chelsea's. Sorry for asking. But yeah, would you? I mean, if you can. I need to get there ASAP, and I'd rather not go alo—"

"I'll be there in twenty minutes. Talk to you then."

I collapse into a chair, sigh in relief, and text Mom: *Will's taking me.*

Twenty minutes later, he shows up wearing khakis and a light-blue button-down cotton shirt. "My standard future-internship outfit. A poor excuse for mourning attire, but it's the best I could do. Sorry."

"I don't think Chelsea will mind. She was a fan of blue." Sitting on the stairs, I extend a hand, and he pulls me up.

"Thank you for coming. My mother won't let me drive, and your sister assured me you'd go. I couldn't have done this alone."

"It's the least I can do with everything you and your parents are doing for my sister."

Hi, I'm Madz. I'm helpless and I hate it. "We can take my car if you want."

"No need. I took off the seat covers I use when I work. We'll be sitting on clean fabric. Your mother would be happy to know I disinfected the cab. I even have hand sanitizer." He holds it up.

I smile and say, "Thank you."

Will's pickup truck is louder than I remember. The creaking and rumbling are dead-air resuscitators. The sounds pound and pound away until Will finally speaks.

"I need to say something, and I hope the timing isn't totally inappropriate," he says.

"Inappropriate timing has become a mutual theme between us. Go ahead and say it."

"I assumed the worst about you when you cut off communication, and I'm sorry for that. I'd been programmed to assume the worst, and it's hard to break old habits. When coaches showed up out of the blue for Gracie, I figured you had something to do with it, but I also figured it was your way of washing your hands of us. Your way of distancing yourself because you'd gotten yourself in too deep. I didn't blame you; I was disappointed. I'd convinced myself you were different." His eyes capture mine. "Turns out I was right. You are different." He smiles. "I'm glad the whole situation's been cleared up, and I hope today's a fresh start."

He shakes his head. "My timing sucks, doesn't it? Today's not exactly the best day to talk about fresh starts."

"Your timing's perfect." Looking out the window, I sigh. "I, obviously, owe you an apology too. I made decisions based on my own incorrect assumptions, which, I hear, my mother explained to you." I glance at him. "I guess we're even."

The engine's creaks and rumbles beat the dead air again.

"Would now be a good time to ask who that's for?" He points to my gift bag.

"It's for Chelsea. I mean her mom."

"Not judging, but I've never heard of a funeral gift."

"Good thing you're not judging." A cringeworthy chuckle escapes my mouth. *Oh no*, he could be offended by my not giving him a gift for his mother's death. I cringe, struggling with the awkwardness I inflicted upon both of us by asking him to take me to a funeral. Offering him an out is the best way to rectify the situation. "If this is too hard for you, I totally understand. You can wait in the truck. You don't have to go in."

Reminding him of his loss, I could be the worst friend in the world. This kind of awkwardness is probably what Lindsey wanted to avoid.

"My being here has nothing to do with what I *have* to do. I *want* to keep you company. To be totally honest, Gracie texted me and said your mother wants me to watch you for any signs of sickness."

"Amazing how quickly my mother networks." I chuckle, relieved more than humored by her messaging him, awkward or not. I could drown at this funeral, in sorrow, anxiety, germs, God knows what. Will is my life preserver.

When we pull up to the funeral home, a guy in a black suit, white shirt, and black tie signals to a parking spot and walks up to us. Will rolls down his window. The guy, holding a funeral flag for the car, tells us we'd better hurry in because the viewing's ending soon.

I gasp. "I thought there was no wake," I tell the mortician guy.

"There wasn't. This viewing is part of the funeral. Like I said, you'd better hurry." He puts the funeral flag on the truck and returns to his original spot by the entrance.

Will hops out of the truck and opens my door. Fear plows through my veins, freezing me still while my heart jackhammers my chest.

"Um, what are we doing?" Will says. "And why are you looking at me like a deer in the headlights?"

"Can I tell you the truth?"

He nods.

"I don't think I can do this." I have some nerve saying those words to him. That's how afraid I am of messing this up. I try to apologize. My throat's so tight I let out a hiccoughing sound instead.

"Take in a deep breath and blow it out. I'm going in with you. Everything will be okay. Besides, your mother told me Chelsea thought you were the bomb. You can't not go in."

I'm the bomb, alright. "I'm glad you and my mom are getting along."

"She's a good lady." He holds out his hand. "C'mon. The viewing is almost over. In and out."

Yea, though I walk through the valley of the shadow of death, I will fear no evil.[1] If I keep telling myself that, maybe I'll believe it. *Nothing here is an actual threat*, I tell my brain, but it's too late. It already sent the message to my heart to resume jackhammering.

The air weighs a ton in the funeral home, and my mask limits ventilation even more. Practically suffocating, I enter the room full of people and watch the floor as Will walks me to the casket. He squeezes my hand, then rests his hand on my back, nudging me to kneel before the casket. He kneels beside me.

I silently recite the Hail Mary but stop halfway through, daring my eyes to climb the side of the casket. I find Chelsea's sweet, sleeping face. *Hi, friend,* I say for us alone to hear.

Hi, friend, she whispers back.

If you see the Light, go to it if you haven't already. You're a butterfly now. You can fly wherever you want, and nothing will hurt you. I'll always be your friend. Thank you for being mine when I really needed one. You take care.

I kiss my fingertips, gently place them on her forehead, and tear up. *Stop it, stop it, stop it,* I tell myself. Will stands, and I follow his lead. I grip his arm and blink, unleashing the waterworks I tried holding back. Will's hand presses gently against my back as I step toward Chelsea's mom, who's standing at the foot of the casket with Chelsea's father. I met him once at the hospital.

They both put on masks. I hug Theresa and say, "I'm so sorry."

"Be happy for her. She's free of that sick little body of hers."

I can be happy Chelsea's out of her sick body, but that doesn't change how depressing it is her body was so sick in the first place. It doesn't change how horrible it must be for her parents to lose their child.

Chelsea's father hugs me. "Thank you for making her last wish come true."

"She was my friend. Speaking of friends, this is Will. My mother got called into work; she was needed at the courthouse."

Theresa nods, smiles at Will, who says, "I'm sorry for your loss." He holds my hand and gently pulls me to the back of the room. The funeral director stands before the casket. Ending the viewing period, he leads us in an Our Father and Hail Mary.

IF THIS WERE a movie depicting a child's funeral, the mood would be set with clouds looming above, siphoning the landscape's color. Instead, the sun-lit sky beams down on a lush landscape, a palette of primary colors and pastels. With one dark smear, the funeral party.

We stand under a tree, a burial location I don't get. Don't the roots interfere with grave digging, and wouldn't they eventually wrap around the casket? I whisper the latter question to Will.

In response, he whispers, "Caskets are put inside cement tombs. Roots shouldn't be an issue. If they do become a problem, Chelsea won't care, so don't worry about it."

As we wait for the minister, a bird chirps relentlessly in what I'm sure is its version of barking—at the dozen geese walking by the grave as if they're overseeing the funeral. Chelsea's younger brother pulls on his mother's dress and points at the scene. She looks, runs her hand over his head, and smiles. Before she slips on her sunglasses, she winks at me.

The minister welcomes the guests and says, "How painful it is to lose a child—a daughter, a sister, a friend . . ." I zone out, absorbing bits of his sermon that translate to: "Our sister Chelsea" is pain-free and with God; we're blessed to have known her; someday we'll reunite with her . . .

I creep away from the crowd so I can take off my mask and suck in the fresh air.

Will wraps his arm around me. "Are you okay?"

A white butterfly lands on the grass by a tree, fluttering its wings as if showing them off to me. "Yeah."

After, we throw roses onto the casket, a process Will walks me through. I've been to exactly one funeral: my grandfather's, two years ago. (I'd've gone to Lindsey's grandmother's if it weren't out of state.) I didn't pay attention to the process because all I had to do was follow the grown-ups. Also handicapping my funeral IQ, my nerves have short-circuited. I'm unable to improvise, can only concentrate on breathing, staying conscious, and containing any cues that would divulge my unraveling. Other than the hand tremor as I drop the rose, I think I'm successful.

We walk to a nearby building, an actual in-cemetery venue, and the weight of the gravesite lifts; my nerves settle. "Wait," I tell Will. "I have to get the gift."

I scurry to the truck, grab the gift, and we return to the venue.

"Whew, cool air," I say, my head overheating under my wig. I'd love to rip it off.

Will and I dig into the homestyle food at our table.

Will cleans his plate. "I don't mean to be disrespectful if that's what this is." He presents his empty plate. "But *mmm*, five stars for cemetery food. Think about it. This is a cemetery restaurant."

A smile erupts on my face, which is in shock because, well, a genuine smile erupted on my face. Theresa catches my eye. I nod, ashamed for smiling. What's wrong with me?

Some people laugh as they pick through the dessert table.

Theresa's husband heads there. I'm about to get up and give her the gift when she walks over to my table.

"How are you?" she asks me. "Are you sick of people asking you that?" This woman must be a saint, asking me how I am, and here comes the weird thing: the second she asks, guess who can't control the waterworks?

"I'm so sorry." My words trip over jerky breaths. "I shouldn't be doing this."

Then guess what? Theresa starts crying.

Will's head ping-pongs from me to her to me again. He hands me his napkin, says, "No, that's dirty," and asks the waitress for some clean napkins.

"Here, I have an endless supply of tissues," Theresa says, handing me one. "I thought I was ready. I know she was." She sighs and shrugs. "Chelsea told me she was ready, and I know she meant it. What six-year-old knows they're ready to go to Heaven?" She pats her eyes with a tissue. "That's the only thing getting me through this."

"I believe her," I say. "I mean, she seemed so tired."

"She was. She'd been sick most of her life. We thought she might beat the odds and outlive the cancer. In another week, she would have turned seven." She rests her hand on my arm. "Oh, but Madz, you have a totally different type of cancer. Your mother told me you're almost done with your treatments." She smiles and silently claps.

Yay, me. I shift in my seat, stirred by guilt. "Tomorrow's my last." How dare I discuss my good news at her daughter's funeral! I hand Theresa a small, sparkly, pink gift bag that one of my Sweet Sixteen gifts came in. I didn't have the heart to get rid of it because *sparkles*.

She pulls out the ornament I bought one summer at a Christmas store near a skating camp I'd attended.

"I know Chelsea shared my affinity for glittery things," I say.

"A cherub. She's beautiful," Theresa says.

"She reminds me of Chelsea." Chubby cheeks, shimmering wings, and her hair is short and curly, how Theresa described Chelsea's pre-chemo hair. "I meant to give it to her when we went to the rink, but I forgot. Chemo fog, I guess."

She cups the cherub in her hand and studies it. "After we visited the butterfly garden, Chelsea told me that when she became an angel, she wanted shimmery wings like the butterfly you showed her." She looks up from it. "Thank you, Madz. I needed this."

We say our goodbyes, and when Will and I go outside, the air is lighter and easier to breathe.

"That was . . . different. In a really . . . good and unexpected way," Will says.

"Different? Try *difficult*."

"Don't get me wrong," he says. "What happened to Chelsea sucks. Nothing's worse than burying a child. But there you were, giving her mother a gift. Unusual, yet it symbolized something special you and Theresa understood about Chelsea, who told her parents she was ready to die. And under their loving watch, she did. Therefore, this funeral was unexpectedly good—different from what I'd expected—because of its sense of closure. For her mother, her father, even you."

"Closure."

"Yeah." He opens the truck door for me. "Everyone's at peace now. Chelsea's no longer suffering; her parents, who knew their daughter's death was imminent, got to hear from Chelsea's own lips she was ready to die, and you have the satisfaction of knowing you broke a gift-giving barrier and made your being there personal. In the end, as tragic as her whole story is, Chelsea got what she wanted, and those she left behind got to say goodbye and have a sense of peace. If you ask me, all involved are lucky in that respect."

He scurries around the truck, into the driver's seat, and we drive off.

"She got ripped off. She only got to live a short time, and that time was spent in a sick body and measured in treatment cycles. A sense of peace doesn't take away how sad that is."

"No, but it takes the edge off. Everyone has a clear conscience. At least her parents and you can have peace of mind knowing you did everything you could to make her happy while she was alive."

Dead air follows his remark. Essentially, he's telling me his conscience isn't clear. He knows his way around a funeral, yet his mother, already cremated, hasn't had a wake or funeral. Hasn't had any acknowledgment of her leaving this world or having lived in it. Her two children prove there must have been a time she truly lived and contributed in a positive way to their upbringing. They're both good people. They had to have had a decent role model at some point early on.

"How did you get so good at funerals?" I ask. "You knew everything to do and when to do it."

His eyes fix on the highway. "Experience. I think one of the reasons why my mother was so, you know, was because her mother, father, and sister died one after the other. Got to the point where all she did was obsess about death and being abandoned by my father."

The road's white lines blur as I search for the right words.

A simple truth comes to mind. "Judging from how you watch out for Gracie and how hard you work, you've been the backbone of your family. It seems to me you did everything you could to make your mother happy. I hope that gives you a sense of peace."

He flashes me an intense glimpse. "I let her down." Looking at the road, he bites his lips. "But it would've been nice if she'd given me a hint her last threat was different."

I sigh, shimmy to the left, as far as my seatbelt will let me move, and rest my hand on his shoulder. "I learned in my psych class that depressed people can plummet into this, like, dark abyss, where their judgment can go off the rails." Basically, what Harper told me. "Let's say she did hint that this time was different, and you were able to prevent her death. What about the next time?

"It's impossible to control someone else's actions. We can only control our own, and you worked, paid the bills, and helped Gracie. You went the extra mile to take any excess weight off your mother's shoulders." My hand slips off his arm and joins my other hand on my lap.

He continues to focus on the road. "When I was at the funeral, I thought my mother was in a weird way like Chelsea. She had a horrible disease she couldn't control and was ready to die. I get that. But Gracie and I were her kids. We should have meant something to her, even in the abyss. If I had kids, I'd never desert them." He throws me another glimpse. "Your parents would never abandon you."

I squirm, his comment having struck a nerve tethered to an angry thought I've suppressed for years. Until now. "My birth mother overdosed on heroin. You'd think she'd want to stay sober for her preschooler, right? She told my mother she was sober while pregnant with me. Kind of like, okay, I did my good deed; now give me my shit. And she took so much it killed her."

"Well, then, I stand corrected." He glances at me. "I'm sorry that happened to you." Eyes on the road, he clenches his jaw and shakes his head. "You should have mattered more to her than getting high, especially because you were so young. Were—are—you mad at her?"

I shrug. "Nah, she was sick, Will. I learned that over time from my mother, who did a good job explaining it. She'd consulted a therapist to prep for our discussions about my adoption and birth mother."

"Yeah, I can see your mother not settling for anything less than an expert briefing covering all the conversational bases of the topic. She's such a lawyer." He chuckles.

"I know, right? Anyway, the therapist told her my birth mother's drive to get her next fix was as strong as the urge to, you know, go to the bathroom when you have a stomach bug. It was an amazing feat she'd stayed sober while pregnant with me. I wasn't born addicted, so at least she did that for me. My biological father just handed over custody. Didn't want anything to do with me. He was pretty sick, too, if you ask me."

He parks in front of my house, unbuckles, and turns to me. He sandwiches my hands between his. "Your biological father put you in the hands of competent parents. At least he did that for you. I'm happy it worked out for you. I really am. My father would take off whenever he pleased and leave Gracie and me with a mother who stuck around physically but was never really there."

He hops out of the truck, opens my door, takes my hand, and helps me out as if fearing I might break. I understand why he might think that. I'm pretty small compared to his truck.

However, with Chelsea's funeral behind me, I'm stronger than earlier. I don't tell him because his touch charges me.

"Thank you," I say, my eyes latching onto his.

"You're welcome. I'm really sorry about Chelsea." He walks me to the front door, his hand on my back.

The physical connection and his gentle demeanor encourage me to return to our conversation about our mothers. "I don't mean to harp, Will, but I think you missed the point I tried to make before mentioning my birth father."

We stop before my front door, and he leans against the house. "You have my full attention. Go ahead and harp." His big, brown eyes home in on mine.

"You and Gracie turned out to be good people despite your mother's flaws. I think if you look hard enough, you'll see that your mother, like my birth mother, had a window of time in which she pushed her demons aside for you and made a positive impression. That's all I'm trying to say. Unfortunately, also like my birth mother, yours lost the battle with those demons."

He straightens his back. "I don't mean to sound mean or ungrateful, but please, do me a favor. Don't try to defend my mother on any level." He looks at his watch. "I gotta go."

And now I've undone everything good about this day.

TWENTY-SEVEN

Mom returns from the courthouse during her lunch break, and I tell her about the funeral and how Will helped me. We go outside, where the sky is hazy, the air humid. She follows me into the gazebo and turns on the fan. It's ten degrees cooler in here; with the fan, even cooler. I cover my legs with my favorite lightweight quilt and sip my iced tea.

"Lindsey still hasn't called or texted me. My friend since childhood hasn't dropped a line in weeks. Nor have my other supposed friends at SuperEdge, except for Joao."

Mom reminds me I'm the one who didn't want to tell anyone about my illness, then she bites into her veggie wrap.

"What does that have to do with it?" I ask her. "Friends text each other. They texted me before I left SuperEdge. Besides, Lindsey knows about my illness and hasn't texted for weeks."

"Have you texted her or any of your friends from the rink besides Joao?" Thus begins the chicken or egg conversation about my skating friends or lack thereof. "It's possible Lindsey and the others think you want nothing to do with them. You made it clear you were done with skating. All they do is skate. When you walked out of the rink, you, at least perceivably, walked out on them. Your not texting them supports that notion. Don't you think?" Another successful case argued by Mom, except for one flaw.

I lie on the couch and adjust the pillow under my head. "I understand why most of the people I skated with might think that way, and I admit I haven't texted any of them. They ignored me at the parking-lot barbecue, simplifying my decision to sever comms. Lindsey's different. She's supposed to be my best friend. Why would she go AWOL?

"If I were in her shoes, I'd think, 'I haven't heard from Madz in a while. Maybe she's super sick.' Then I'd send me an uplifting emoji or meme. Multiple choice question: (a) my cancer scared her away, (b) she thinks she's too good for me, (c) she's afraid of associating with a rink rebel now that Nathan's her coach, or (d) all of the above?"

"I stink at multiple-choice questions. Scooch over." Mom sits beside me. "Lindsey knows about the time you taught Gracie at the rink. Hasn't she connected the dots between you, Nathan, and Gracie? Does she think it's a coincidence? Little does she know, associating with you would get her *into* Nathan's good graces." Mom smirks and checks her texts.

"You're being catty. Shame on you." I smile myself, relieved Nathan helped us instead of blocking us.

"For the record, Lindsey's mother hasn't texted me in weeks." Mom looks up from her phone. "You know, Madz, life gets busy. It wraps people up in routines just as it wrapped us up in ours. It is what it is." She kisses my head, says, "I have to get back to work," and leaves.

The skaters' schedules at SuperEdge are as full as mine used to be. Yet we texted each other back then. The reality is we have nothing in common anymore, and I'm a perceived liability. Two safe-to-assume factors in the no-text equation. I do wonder which of my former friends would pull a Lindsey and which would care, like Joao and Nathan, if they knew about my cancer.

I would have never guessed Nathan and Joao would be more supportive than Lindsey. Joao knows I'm sick and knows about my stormy departure from SuperEdge. Still, he's all in with communicating with me and helping Gracie. No apparent ulterior motives. For God's sake, I walked out on Nathan publicly, and he's still around. Gracie is the glue holding us together, making us think beyond our own selfish realms.

Come to think of it, Gracie is the glue that holds Will and me together. For a moment, I thought he and I connected on a more personal level, but my blabbering shrink-talk annoyed him, possibly digging an emotional moat between us.

Welcome to another episode of Madz Monroe's Pity Party, where I'm the only guest. My judgment about people and etiquette sucks. I shut out people who actually cared about me. I annoyed Will with a loquacious autopsy of his mother's psyche. I scolded my mother for feeling sad about my diagnosis. My parents adopted a dud.

I yawn, stretch, roll over on my side, and curl up like a fetus. I click on my soothing-rain playlist, pull my quilt up to my chest, and drift off to sleep.

RAKING, raking, raking, such a satisfying sound. The earth's getting a good scratching. *Raking in the rain?* I open my eyes to dim sunlight sifting through the gazebo's screen. The sun burned off the haze. I check the time and realize I've slept for almost two hours, and it's not raining. I shut off my soothing-rain sounds playlist and crane my head out, periscoping the yard until I find Will.

I pull the covers over my head, ashamed of being a lazy loser while he's working. The raking closes in. "I know you're awake," he says. "I saw you looking."

Double that loserdom.

"Fine," he says. "Stay under there. I just wanted to say I'm sorry for snapping at you. You tried to make me feel better, and I was rude. I admit when I'm wrong, and that was wrong." More raking.

My head turtles out of my quilt shell. "You weren't rude. You were being honest. I just suck at saying the right thing. I'm the one who should be sorry." I fold down my quilt to waist level, relieved I didn't offend him. "Sorry."

He stops raking, sits on a step outside the gazebo, and stares at the pool.

"You can sit in here, you know," I say. "It's cool under the fan."

"Maybe another time. I'm shedding dirt and grass. I thought about what you said about my mother. I went way back to before my father started going out drinking every night, before he started gambling away our money. When we lived in a nice house like yours. My father used to tell me to go to college and learn about money. 'Become an investment banker,' he'd say. I'd tell him, 'Okay,' but then tell my mother I wanted to plant flowers. Make every yard as nice as ours."

He turns to me. "I couldn't stand seeing a messy yard, knowing how good it could look."

"No judgment. I have a similar affliction."

"So did my mother, but she preferred planting to pulling weeds, which I got stuck doing. That's why I charge a premium for it." He chuckles. "She always involved me in the yard work. We were a team. When I was little, she bought me a toy lawn mower for Christmas, and being the little ingrate I was, I cried because it didn't actually cut grass. So when I was twelve, just before my father lost his job, she bought me a real lawn mower. She said, 'My one wish for you is whatever you do, you'll be happy doing it.'

"Then our world crumbled down on us, and my father's girlfriend was one of the cockroaches who came out of the woodwork. Along with some guy who said he now owned the title to our house. My mother said she could live with being poor, but living with a broken heart was murder. Nevertheless, the moral to this story is yes, there was a moment in time my mother did something selfless and motherly. Thank you for pointing that out to me."

"Her illness may have gotten the best of her," I say, "but I knew she had to be a good person. You and Gracie have work ethics, a good sense of right and wrong, and you're both caring people. It takes some degree of character honing as a child to acquire those qualities."

I'm relieved he recalled positive memories of his mother, flowers among the weeds. He can replay the sweet treasures in his mind whenever he needs an emotional boost. "I'd help you landscape if I weren't out of commission."

"It's just a moment in time, right? Before you know it, you'll be up and running, on your way to college and a new life."

His pep talk sounds like a breakup. How can we break up when we haven't had a chance to be together? I sit up. "I don't want a new life. Just a healthier one."

He looks at his watch. "I have to pick up Gracie from camp."

"Can I go with you, or are you sick of driving me around?"

"I put the crappy covers back on the seats. You'll get dirty. Your mother will freak."

"Let's take my car. I'll drive." I miss driving. One normal thing. The thought of doing it energizes me. The thought of spending more time with him does too.

"I thought you were afraid because of what happened. Sorry. I don't mean to rehash it, but your mother told me how sick you were the day you came to visit Gracie at the rink."

"I won't be afraid if you're with me, and as long as you're in the car, my mother would be okay with it." I pull the gazebo's screen curtain aside and poke my head out. "Do I sound too clingy?"

"You sound like you're trying to regain your independence, and I'm sort of like your training wheels."

"Ugh, really? I'm sorry." I'm doomed to sabotage my relationship with this guy.

"Sorry for what? I'm glad you feel safe with me."

I smile, savoring the sweetness of his comment. I step out of the gazebo and catch a glimpse of the lawn surrounding the poolhouse. Pure lawn. "Where are all the dandelions?"

He turns toward the poolhouse. "You're a fan of them all of a sudden? I pulled them."

"I didn't think my parents noticed how out of control they got. They've been so busy. I'm glad they finally paid you to clear them out of there."

He looks at me. "They didn't. I figured you might not have the energy to battle them, so I dug them up, root and all. They won't harass you again."

"You did that for me?"

He nods, holds me with his eyes, and warm waves roll through my body. Our relationship has officially progressed to the next level.

I DROP Gracie off at the rink for her lesson with Joao. She runs in, needing to change into her skating clothes before her lesson. I park the car and ask Will, "Can I watch her for five minutes? I know you have to get back to work."

"I do. I have three more yards to do. But work's a wash till Gracie's done with her lesson. I'd have to get back here by the time I got to the job."

Walking into the rink, I worry a microbe will dive into my lungs and make me sick again. I worry even though my doctor reassured me I was sick before setting foot in here. Will and I stand by a small section of the boards with no acrylic glass between our eyes and the skaters.

I zip my jacket and hug myself as Gracie strokes around the rink. My mask creates a weak barrier between the cold and my face. Will rests his sweatshirt over my shoulders, leaving his arm around me.

Joao skates to the boards. "As soon as Will leaves, she'll get testy with me." He's wearing a down coat, a scarf, and a winter beanie.

"A beanie? I never thought I'd see the day you squash your hair," I say.

"This rink is freezing."

"You, Nathan, and Lindsey cleaned up her technique," I say.

"Trust me, it wasn't easy with those skates. Take a good look at her feet. She pronates. A solid boot and arch support would correct that."

"I've had to buy her used skates," Will says. "Her feet grow so fast—at least, they did—and I have a budget. New skates cost a fortune. Why couldn't she pick a less expensive sport like badminton?"

When Mom took Gracie to get her skates sharpened, my skate guy traced Gracie's foot, saying he wanted to make sure her current skates were the right size. He was really sizing her for a new pair. I'd tell Will about the surprise, but I'm afraid he might get offended if I say it in front of Joao.

"They're a good brand of skates. I've seen a lot worse," I say.

Gracie stops by Joao. "Show your brother and Madz a clean waltz-loop-loop combination," Joao says. Gracie does a waltz jump only, holds up a wait-a-minute index finger, does a waltz jump, a loop, holds her back edge in preparation for another loop . . .

Her ankle gives out, and she slips off her edge. Her cheeks flush, and she bites her lips as she skates toward Joao. She's winding up for it; I can tell.

Joao doesn't budge from his spot. His coaching style reminds me of Nathan's. Ha. *Watch out, Gracie, you're in for some competition.* Instead of screaming, she lets out a short, loud grunt. While skaters roll their eyes (one snarls) in response, Joao grunts back at Gracie. Loudly.

"Quiet," the proctor says, her microphoned voice echoing throughout the rink.

I'm stunned to see Gracie slide down against the boards to a sitting position and laugh. Joao reaches his hand out to her, she takes it, and he pulls her up. "Tighten your laces." She skates to the penalty box.

"I read that some kids on the autism spectrum are sensitive to loud sounds," I say.

"True," Will says. "Maybe the noise doesn't bother them when they're making it."

"I don't think her little hissy fits have anything to do with her autism issues," Joao says, signaling Gracie to skate back to him.

"I'm impressed," Will says. "How long did it take you to figure that out?"

"By our second lesson, when I realized she was a control-freak perfectionist like Nathan. I think she low-key channels him. Only Nathan's a silent screamer, which is way scarier."

"Yes, definitely," I say. "Brilliant analysis, by the way."

Gracie laces her skates quickly and snugly, surprising me.

"She's gotten better at tying," I say to Will.

"Joao has that effect on her," he says. "It also helps that she's been practicing for years. It finally paid off."

Gracie returns to Joao, who sends her off to try the waltz-loop-loop combination again. She skates around, picks up speed, and performs the jump successfully.

Will and I clap, and I let out a "Whoo-hoo! Good job, Gracie."

"Nathan informed me she has to take her freestyle test on Sunday at ten a.m.," Joao says, handing Will a test form. "We need your signature. Nathan took care of the fee."

"Why rush her freestyle test?" Will asks, signing the form.

"A lot of reasons," Joao says. "Nathan re-evaluated her the other day and decided she was ready. Her loop will be consistent as long as her skates are laced snugly and her blades are sharp. She's pretty determined, so nerves shouldn't be an issue. The test will be a good warm-up for ice-theater auditions, which, I hate to tell you, were pushed up to Sunday afternoon. If she passes the test, she'll go into theater tryouts with confidence.

"If she doesn't pass the test, she's still almost guaranteed a spot on the ice-theater team. She's got the talent and drive, and Nathan put in a good word for her. One way or another, she'll have a good day Sunday."

"Thank you, Joao," Will says. He takes money out of his pocket. "What do I owe Nathan for the test?"

Joao holds up his hand, refusing Will's money. "He said it was a gift." He tucks his hands into his pockets. "She only has to pay him back if she fails."

I gasp.

"Just kidding," Joao says. "But for real, Nathan said it was taken care of." Gracie skates up to him. "Do a back scratch spin, then skate a lap and try a flip." He turns to Will. "If you're itching to get rid of money, I'll take a few bucks for gas. I need it to get to her test. My parents aren't as rich as this chick's over here." He thumbs in my direction.

Will hands him money. "Here's the thirty-five dollars I would have used to pay for the test. Thanks, Joao."

I nudge Will. "Cheaper than what it cost you for my test."

He nudges me. "And less of a fiasco." He tells Joao, "I'm sure I owe you a lot more for the lessons."

"You owe me nothing. You can pay me for lessons after I

get her through this test and ice-theater tryouts. I want to prove myself as a coach first. To Nathan *and* Gracie."

I hug Joao. "I had no idea what a doll you are. Thank you."

Gracie checks out of a slow, centered back scratch spin. She skates around the rink and does a flip. Will and I clap, then we each give her a thumbs-up. Joao skates up to Gracie and high-fives her.

Because twenty minutes remain in the session and I'm freezing, Will buys me a hot chocolate in the lame café. "Do you think it's safe?" I ask.

"The water's boiled. Any bugs in it are dead."

"That's what I was thinking." I blow on it, unable to drink it until it's almost room temperature. Hot chocolate is a double-edged sword for me. It's a good choice for warming me up, a bad choice for my chemo throat.

We leave the café at the sound of the end-of-session buzzer. The proctor stomps up to Will, her cheeks flaming red. "I warned your sister last week about her yelling. I let her skate here this week, and she thanked me by grunting. Her behavior is unacceptable. We have coaches out there trying to give lessons and skaters trying to concentrate. They've put up with enough." She glares at Will. "And now her coach is making funny sounds. Take your sister and her coach to another rink."

"You'd be doing Gracie a favor if you did, Will. C'mon." I take his arm.

"No!" Gracie says, crying in the doorway, standing with Joao behind the lady.

"Chill, Gracie. She's just being a fart," Joao says.

Gracie erupts with giggles. She leaves with Joao and Will. "I'll be right there," I say to them.

"Excuse me," I say to the proctor. "I'm sorry if Joao and

Gracie caused a disruption. But in case you didn't notice, Gracie's *one singular* grunt this session was shorter and far less loud than her previous yelps. Joao helped Gracie by being silly. Your skaters could help too. Maybe if they said hi to Gracie once in a while instead of snarling and rolling their eyes at her, she'd want to be more considerate."

"You shouldn't blame others for her behavior."

"I'm not. I'm speaking the truth. Gracie has improved, yet your skaters are still making faces at her. One almost ran over her while she was setting up for her loop. I didn't hear the skater warn Gracie, and I didn't hear you warn the careless skater. I don't mean to be disrespectful. I just don't think Gracie's being treated fairly."

"See how well she's treated if she skates at SuperEdge. They wouldn't have half the patience these skaters and I have had."

I step back three feet and pull my mask down. "Sorry Gracie made your lives so miserable. Personally, I love seeing someone who cares about skating so much that she gets frustrated if she thinks she failed at it. And just so you know, Gracie's mother died this week. The last thing she needs is dirty looks from fellow skaters. I happen to know SuperEdge does have her back. Where do you think her coach is from?"

"He's from SuperEdge?"

"Have a nice day." I pocket my mask and bolt to the car.

I guarantee her skaters and their mothers would be nice to Gracie if they knew her connections to SuperEdge Skating Club. I huff in frustration, upset over the nasty looks skaters here gave Gracie, upset at myself for having been like them the first time I met her, upset over a grown adult being so harsh. All of us are too imperfect to be snobs. Some kids express themselves with a shrill instead of a whimper. We should be able to handle the mild discomfort of a yelp emitted by a kid suffering extraordinary circumstances.

On the way home, Will drives. I roll down my window, hold down my wig, and breathe in the warm, fresh air. He takes an unexpected turn, stopping at a small park on the opposite side of town from where I live. The lot's near low-income housing and had once been home to a small municipal building. I know because my father thought of buying it. His excuse for not buying it was "Too much red tape. I'd have to build what they wanted me to build." The building was torn down; the lot, neglected. Until now.

"It's beautiful," I say. "A far cry from the eyesore that was there."

"Will made that," Gracie says.

"You did?" I ask him.

"Yeah," Gracie says. "It was his contest entry, and he won."

"The sectioned-off plots are for community farming and educating kids in the neighborhood about horticulture. I rigged solar-powered, self-irrigation systems for each plot." He also paved a few paths. One leads to a terraced sitting area with a tiny library.

"It's beautiful," I say.

"The teacher in the woodworking shop at school helped me build the little house for books. We shingled it and everything."

A pot of perennials decorates a spot near the entrance. "I love the bold colors," I say. "Is that your work too?" I point to the pot.

"Yeah. The city said they'd pay me to maintain it and allow me to put up a small sign to advertise my business. Not much, but something. And they gave me a small budget to make it season friendly. Next month I'll decorate it with hay bales, pumpkins, and a scarecrow. See the hill over there?"

"Yeah."

"I built it so kids could slide down it when we have snow. For now, they can climb up the hill and roll down. Basic stuff they couldn't do before with all the concrete surrounding them. The extra space near it is so they can kick a ball around."

"There's a purpose for every space, and it's community friendly," I say. "It's an urban oasis. If just one detail weren't there, it wouldn't be so . . . perfect. Gracie said you didn't train in landscaping; you're just really good at it. She's right."

"I did train. My shop teacher got me a landscaping job with his friend when I was fourteen. It was part of a special work program I'd applied for. I learned everything I could for two years, then started my own business. I needed more money, and my boss wasn't paying enough. Anytime I had questions about irrigation, paving, masonry, electrical—anything—I'd ask the appropriate teacher after school. Some had side jobs in their trades, and they'd let me come with them and watch. So although I appreciate my sister's take on my talent, a lot of people helped me get good at it."

I want to do something similar someday. Design the layout of schools, housing complexes, public gardens. Reconfigure cityscapes to fit in more agriculture zones. "I love the idea of injecting life into otherwise dead, concrete spaces. Especially when so many people live in those spaces."

"Let's go, guys. This is boring," Gracie says.

As Will drives to my house, he says, "Those patches of life can be a godsend to some people. I think that's why I'm drawn to landscaping. Surrounding myself with living, growing things and all their colors and scents always lifted me up, especially after spending a night in my apartment, surrounded by sadness."

"Nothing beats the smell of life," I say. Beats the smell of cooked eggs and canned tuna.

"I wish I could do more urban-renewal projects. I'll get the opportunity to during my internship, but I had to put that job on hold until after fall cleanup. Makes more financial sense for me, and I don't want to lose my customers for an internship that doesn't guarantee future employment."

He turns into my driveway, I click open the garage, and he drives in. He hops out of the car and runs to my side even though I've already opened my door. He holds out his hand for me.

I'd love to grab it but don't want to take advantage of his chivalry. "I'm fine now that I made it through Chelsea's funeral, but thank you," I say, getting out of the car.

"I can tell you're fine," he says, standing close. "I thought I'd hold your hand anyway. If that's okay."

I smile and reach for his hand. Holding it grounds me in the world of the living and reassures me he forgives me for leaving him and Gracie in the dark about my illness. When he interlocks his fingers with mine as we walk to his truck, he convinces me he's willing to give himself a chance at being happy despite his mother's death.

"You're being goofy, Will," Gracie says from the garage.

"It's okay; I like goofy," I say, my eyes trapped in Will's.

Gracie runs into the house. Will stops short of his truck and says, "Hey. Your mother told me you were afraid to tell Gracie and me you were sick. Can I ask why it was so hard to tell us?"

"It wasn't just you and Gracie. I didn't want anyone to know. I was afraid people would assume I was doomed, and I was afraid of being treated differently. I feared being pitied, presumed terminal, things like that. Now, at the tail end of this disaster, I don't care who knows. I just don't want cancer to define me."

"Wow."

"What?"

"I get it. That's exactly how I feel about . . ."

"You can say it. You're—ugh. There I go again." I want to reassure him he's already defined himself. I also want to hug him, tell him my heart aches for him, but why cast upon him what I'd feared people would cast upon me, pity?

"There's not much to talk about anymore regarding my mother or the entire tragic story of my family life. It's a done deal. She made a choice to check out, my father made his choices, and I'm making mine. I won't let their choices define me."

"I wish you could come in and watch a movie with me."

"I'd love to, but time is money, and I have to finish work before it gets dark." He looks down the street, his silence telling me he's lost in a place far beyond the road.

"You're not alone, Will." My mirror taught me how to recognize a person in need of those words. They aren't heavy lifters, but they can lighten the load.

He sighs. "I know." He pecks my forehead. "I'll talk to you later, okay?" Heading to his truck, he slouches like he did the first time I noticed the world's weight on his shoulders.

I'd give anything to know the perfect words to say, words capable of lifting the tonnage off of him. My heart's telling me no words can hoist that kind of weight. Only time can.

TWENTY-EIGHT

The dustification of Will's mother happens the same day chemo ravages my body for the last time. Nothing. No. Thing. Comes between this necessary evil and my puking in response to it. Candy brings me a barf bag in preparation for what she's grown to expect. Primed with my nausea medicine, I hold out hope, however frivolous, that this time will be different and the medicine will work.

With every hurl, I beg my body to never relapse. With every hurl, I imagine the Red Devil as a fierce warrior tossing grenades at cancer cells or cells threatening to turn cancerous. With every hurl, I see and smell the mayo-steeped tuna sandwich from two weeks ago. Worsening the shitstorm, the fire in my throat has me fighting off images of what's happening to Will's mother's body today.

Cancer, death, fire. The images swirl in my head like a whirlpool, agitating the raging beast squeezing my stomach, pushing bile up my ulcerated throat. *Think of good things*, I beg myself.

I imagine breathing in the aroma of fresh-cut grass. The smell of my yard after it rains. The lavender by the gazebo. Clean scents and bright colors, even those of dandelions. And then I see a glowing sun at the end of a dark road.

There's an end to this, and I'm almost there, I tell myself. Also encouraging, I won't receive bleomycin.

When the puking finally stops, I rinse my mouth with cool water and suck on a frozen fruit pop to soothe the ulcers in my mouth.

Candy pumps me up with 250 cc of IV fluid to replace what I've lost. She delivers my other infusions, and after the last goes in, she disconnects me from my line and says, "Congratulations. You did it." She high-fives me with her gloved hand. "How's the nausea?"

I wiggle my hand, signaling *eh*, my throat too sore to form words.

The nurse and Mom walk me to the bell, where Dad and Gallagher wait for me, Dad holding a "Congratulations" balloon. Mom kisses my head and nudges me toward the bell. Gallagher takes a picture of me ringing it and a shot of my parents and me by the bell. Then a nurse takes a picture of me, my parents, and Gallagher together by the bell. All the while, one part of me feels as though I'm rubbing my achievement in Chelsea's face. Another part experiences the relief associated with waking from a nightmare.

I'm done with chemo.

Candy tells me the smoldering sores in my esophagus and on my tongue will heal within two weeks. Basically, I'm a walking, talking, simmering log after a forest fire.

Dad returns to work, and Gallagher, Mom, and I go home. Gallagher lets me ride shotgun. I recline the seat, a tattered remnant of a person with a window view of life flashing by. Tired and weak, I'm not ready to hop on that train. Even if I were ready, I wouldn't know my destination.

When I reached for the bell at the clinic, I hesitated. *What now?* I thought. The world's been working, going to school, creating, living. I've been carted around, showing up for treatments, and battling side effects. I never got the chance to learn who I am outside the rink. Now, I don't know who I am outside the hospital. I'm too weak to teach skating or to landscape, and on what resumé is surviving several rounds with the Red Devil relevant experience?

Mom drives by Will's project.

"Stop," I say to her.

She pulls over.

"Will did that," I say, pointing. I open the door and, to protect myself from the sun, pull my cotton hoodie over my head. "Come with me."

"Keep the air conditioning on, please," Gallagher says. "I'll admire Will's work from here."

Mom and I walk along a narrow path and sit on a bench near the tiny library. "Look." I point to the small plaque on a nearby boulder. It reads:

"'Urban Oasis' by Will Cruz. Winner of the Third Annual CitySpark Landscaping Competition."

"We'll have to come back and add a few books to the library," Mom says.

Sitting there, in the middle of what Will created, warm waves roll through me again, powered by a swarm of butterflies.

A car honks, and a truck's engine roars when a red light

changes to green. My eyes dart to Mom's car to see if Gallagher's okay. He waves to me.

"We have to pick up Gracie from camp," Mom says. "Will's . . . busy. I'll drop Gallagher off at home on our way."

"Is she skating today?"

"No."

"We should do something special for Will and Gracie. We could have a ceremony for their mother here." I douse my burning throat with ice water. "She ended her life, but that doesn't mean her life didn't matter. I mean, look at this. She raised a son who built this."

Mom surveys Will's creation. "Whether he did this or not, she deserves a special ceremony to honor her life. It could help Will and Gracie too. Grieving with friends and family could jumpstart the healing process. I just don't want to push them. They've been through enough. Let's follow Will's lead and do whatever we can to help."

GRACIE SITS QUIETLY in the back seat until we pass a random street. "Turn here," she says.

"I can't," Mom says. "I have to go back to my office for a couple of hours."

Gracie's face reddens, and her eyes fill up. "Then drop me off right there." She points to a street corner.

"I'm in charge of keeping you safe," Mom says. "I can't drop you off anywhere."

"I walked home from there by myself before. I need to get home. I need to go in and see—"

"I'll take you tomorrow, honey," Mom says, interrupting Gracie. "Then we won't have to rush."

Gracie covers her head with her arms and rocks, panting out breaths that sound like loud shushes. After a series of right turns, Mom stops before an old two-family house on a street lined with battered multifamily homes. Unlike the others, this house has had a facelift. It's neatly painted in gray with white trim. Flower boxes filled with pink and white impatiens decorate the sturdy porch, before which a perfectly manicured emerald lawn carpets the small front yard. Will's signature.

Gracie jumps out, runs up the stairs, opens the door, and runs up a flight of stairs inside the house. Mom and I rush out of the car and stand on the porch.

"Oh no, the door is locked!" Gracie hollers from the top of a staircase.

Mom eyes me. "Text Will and tell him to get here if he can."

An elderly woman comes out of the first-floor apartment as Gracie comes down the stairs.

Mom's brows curl up, and she slowly shakes her head. "Why did I do this?" she mumbles. "She's still in denial about her mother."

My phone buzzes with a response. "Will says he's on his way," I tell her in a low voice.

"Do you have the key?" Gracie asks the lady.

"I do have the key, dear, but I can't let all of you in without Will being here." I assume this petite, gray-haired woman is the landlady.

"I want to see my mother," Gracie says. "Let me in. C'mon, Mrs. Truman." She waves her hand toward Mom and me. "They can wait here."

"Your mother's not up there, Gracie," Mrs. Truman says. "I'm sorry."

"How do you know?" Gracie asks. "Did you go inside?"

She winces and eyes Mom. "The police told me. I'm sorry, dear. I'm so sorry."

She's a good liar. I admire her ability to exercise common sense under the circumstances. She's entangled in Gracie's stare, and this poor woman found Mrs. Cruz, details of which must be flashing through her head.

After almost ten minutes of Gracie pleading with Mrs. Truman and Mom prodding Gracie to leave, Will pulls up. He runs to Gracie. "C'mon." He holds her hand and takes her upstairs to their apartment. He leaves her there and runs back downstairs to the porch. "You guys can go. Thanks for texting me, Madz."

Mom and I look at each other. Will juggles landscaping jobs and parenting his sister. Now, he's forced to tend to her psychological needs while sifting through remnants of his mother's life, separating the keepers from the weeds. I don't know how he stays as strong as he does.

"Don't look so worried, you two," he says. "Everything's okay. I'll have Gracie back at your house in an hour. I'm sorry about the drama." He runs up the stairs.

TWENTY-NINE

Gallagher hands me ginger ale in a chilled glass because he's that awesome. I pull off my wig, cover my head with my soft cotton beanie, and beeline it to the gazebo, dousing the flames in my throat with a few sips of my cool drink. No quilt for me today. I turn on the fan and pass out on the couch.

I WAKE up at 5:30 p.m., two hours after I fell asleep. Water babbling prompts me to check my phone. As I suspected, I never turned on my soothing-sounds playlist. The gentle splashing charms me off the couch, into the yard, to a three-tiered stone fountain in a shady nook. A tiny fairy sits on each tier, and a pink, glittery ribbon wraps around the base. I reach for the card tucked behind the bow.

"Belated Happy Birthday, and congratulations on finishing

your treatments. Love, Will and Gracie." I sit on the grass next to my fountain, relishing the cool stone ridges my fingers slip down before dipping into the water. When you're as sick as I've been, small things, like the sound and feel of this fountain, are huge.

Hope flickers inside me as I lie on the grass, close my eyes, and listen to the babbling. Hope that despite the major pitfalls of this summer, Will, Gracie, and I will find our way back to normal lives, if normal is even a real thing.

"Do you like it?" Gracie says. "The fairies were my idea."

I open my eyes, shade them out of habit, and find her staring down at me. "I love it, especially the fairies." I'm so relieved she's okay.

"They're magical."

She joins me on the grass, lying a foot away from me on the right, a foot too close, but I'll survive. Magical fairies have my back.

"I think you're right. They remind me of the fairies I saw at Fairies and Such Butterfly Garden with my friend Chelsea. You should come with me sometime." I unshade my eyes and stare at the sky because I can. The sun is falling on the opposite side of the arborvitaes shading me. "You and Will did a good job setting this up for me. It must have been hard for you to decorate it after what happened today."

The area has been covered with a tarp for the past two weeks. Mom told me our electrician was building a lamppost.

"I got over it. Besides, Will put the bow on. I can't believe you didn't wake up when we uncovered it. It made a lot of crinkly noises, and then Will whisper-yelled at me when I almost ran into the gazebo because a bee was chasing me."

I giggle. "I hate when bees chase me."

Staring at the sky, Gracie sighs. "I told my mother to come see me skate sometime, but instead, she killed herself. She didn't care about me and Will enough to stay alive."

She was too sick. She couldn't help it. I'd say the words if I thought they'd make a difference. I hold her hand and track the honking geese flying by in V-formation. As they disappear into the horizon, the trickling fountain calms the air again.

"We both hit rock bottom this summer, Gracie. The good thing about that? Things can only get better from here."

The grass rustles from footsteps. Gallagher's. He grunts and *Ows* as he journeys to supine position a few feet to my left. I peek at him before resting my eyes back on the sky. He's looking up too. Until now, I never imagined the depth of pain he must have experienced from losing his son and daughter-in-law. All the years he worked for my family, he must have longed for his the way Gracie longs for her mother. The way I long for my health and once longed for a mother I lost but never truly had.

"Do you think my mother is up there, Gallagher?" Gracie asks.

"She's everywhere now, like my son and Madzy's birth mother." He looks at me and smiles, then his eyes return to the sky with mine. "Everything's going to be just fine, Miss Gracie. So don't you worry, lass."

A moment passes.

"What the heck is a lass?" Gracie says. Then something weird happens. All three of us burst out laughing—body-quaking, tears-streaming-down-our-faces laughing.

I roll on my side, holding my stomach. After all the weeks of puking, it's about to burst from laughter. Rolling onto my back again, I'm surprised to find Will standing over us, staring. His glassy eyes tell me he's been crying. Gracie, Gallagher, and I sweep the laughing tears off our faces and stand.

"Supper will be ready in five minutes," Gallagher says, heading for the house.

"I take it you like the fountain?" Will says.

Smiling, I hug him as tightly as my strength allows. As he hugs me back, Gracie hugs us. Then sorrow burrows into my heart, and I weep for them, for me, for Gallagher, and for all of the people who left us. The Emotional Roller Coaster can't compete with The Life and Times of Madz Monroe.

Minutes later, we go into the house and help Gallagher set the table. Mom and Dad enter the kitchen with a bouquet of "Congratulations" balloons and a cake. My gut twinges, telling me this is disrespectful to Gracie and Will. Yet, they're smiling and helping my parents tie the balloons around the kitchen. Also, Will agrees to stay for dinner.

While everyone eats Gallagher's Irish lasagna, I eat vanilla ice cream.

"I see you're still extremely daring with your flavor choices," Will says.

"Vanilla ice cream is a matter of survival at this point."

"Not for long," Mom says, bringing out the cake, which says *Congratulations, Madz.* "We've reached the light at the end of a pitch-black tunnel. Tonight we leave that dark pit behind us and celebrate the happiness our futures hold."

Normally, I'd cringe at Mom's corniness. This time, I catch Will's eye and grin, knowing our lives could use an injection of corny.

Dad places a gift on the table.

"Ooh," Gracie says.

"It's for you," Mom tells Gracie.

She jerks her head back. "Today isn't my birthday."

She looks at Will, who shrugs.

"When we asked Madz last month what she wanted for her birthday," Mom says, "this was it. They took a while to come in." Mom hands the gift to Gracie. "Open it."

Gracie's eyes widen as she peels the paper off the box. "Skates," she says. "New skates, Will!" She opens the box, holds one up, and studies it as I did mine the day I left Super-Edge: like it's a precious gem on display at Tiffany's. "I bet I can do an Axel in these."

Mom and I smile at each other.

"I bet you'll pass your freestyle test in those too," I say to Gracie. "You've worked really hard. I know you'll do well."

"I think I'll test in my old skates. At least I know how those work."

"We have an appointment tomorrow morning with the skate guy. He'll heat those and get them to mold to your foot so they're nice and comfortable for your test."

Will squirms in his seat. "How about a thank you, Gracie." His eyes jump from me to my parents. "This is too generous. I'll pay you back, Mr. and Mrs. Monroe." He stands. "I have to get back to work. Thank you for dinner and for giving my sister such a generous gift. Gracie, don't forget to show everyone that thing I emailed you."

"I'll get my laptop."

While Gracie runs upstairs, Mom tells Will, "Please don't pay us back. Maybe it's selfish of us, but giving Gracie those skates makes us happy. We hope it helps you out as well.

You've worked so hard for your family. I don't know anyone else your age who's taken on such a huge responsibility. I told Gracie she has the best brother in the world." She hugs Will. "I appreciate you two being such good friends to my daughter."

I walk him to his truck. "Are you okay? I'm sorry you had to sit through a celebration after you and Gracie had such a rough day."

"I'd saved money to buy her new skates. I had to use it for the . . . you know."

We insulted him. And we took away the joy he would have gotten from giving his sister new skates. No clear line exists between a good deed and insulting a person. Must everything in life be so complicated?

"Hey." He gently lifts my chin with his finger. "No pitying each other, right? Gracie's needs are more important than my ego, so thank you. Your parents paid for them, but it was your birthday wish. I'm grateful. What bothers me? I've already been wondering if I'm enough of a parent for Gracie."

A lock of hair dangles over his forehead. I finger-comb it back into place and say, "You're as good a parent as the best. But it's okay to take a break when you have reliable help. I wish you could've taken the night off of work."

"Work takes my mind off things."

"Maybe sometime I can occupy your mind for a while." After battling cancer and witnessing one kid lose her life and two kids lose their mother, being romantically assertive is ice cream.

He kisses my forehead, hops into his truck, and drives away. I sit on the front steps, my mind a worn but determined broom, sweeping through sadness to clear a path for hope. My family has done everything for me. I can't imagine life without one of my parents or Gallagher. Yet here's Will, on his way to stock shelves for people who have no idea how amazing he is and what he's gone through.

In spite of Will and Gracie's struggles, they know who they are and what they want to do. Gallagher and Nathan have gotten through their trials with strong identities. And Chelsea, weak as she was, kept a grip on hers even in the face of death. Their fortitude inspires me, fueling my flicker of hope into a steady glow. It reassures me I'll write my own story of perseverance, that I'll heal and discover who I am and my purpose on Earth.

Once recovered, I'll exercise my freedom with urgency, knowing setbacks are like waves; they forever roll in. It's only a matter of time before one curls around me again and drags me into the Sea of Unforeseen Circumstances. "Come in, Madz," Mom says.

I go inside and sit next to Gracie at the table. She opens the file Will emailed her. "Will thinks it's safe to show you now." She presses play.

"Marilyn Monroe," the announcer from my test says.

"You're kidding me," Mom says, hovering over my shoulder.

"Exactly what I thought while standing there, posing," I say.

"Sorry. Madelyn Monroe," the announcer says.

"This is your test," Mom says, putting on her readers. "Look, honey," she says to my father, who also dons his readers. "Will videoed this? How?"

"No idea. The first time I saw him that day was after the test, in the parking lot." I look up at her. "He gave me a rose."

"Sweet." She gasps. "Your jumps. They're huge. No one would guess how sick you were."

"The ice was good. Helping matters, I only had to do a single axle and doubles otherwise. No triples."

She blots her eyes. "What a gorgeous spiral."

Gracie, who's clearly seen it before, mimics my arm movements and singles her floor versions of my jumps. Then she holds on to the back of a chair with her leg up, re-enacting my spiral. "The night before your test, I showed Will your internet videos. He said it would be sad if you didn't have a video of your last test." She lets go of the chair, tilts, and grabs hold of it again.

"Keep your tongue in your mouth when you balance, Gracie," Mom says. "If you fall, you could bite it off."

"That's so morbid, Mrs. M.," Gracie says.

"She thinks if she says her sick thoughts out loud, they won't happen," I tell Gracie. I adjust her position, pushing up her free leg. "Point your toe." I place my hand under her jaw. "Chin up."

Mom rewinds the video. "I know I already said this, but your spiral was beautiful, Madz. Wait." She pauses it and studies the image. "Were you . . ."

"Crying. Yes, she was," Gracie says. "See?" She points to the frozen image of my face. "That's a tear."

"I wasn't crying," I say. "One measly tear slipped out."

Mom buries her face in her hands. Dad rubs her back.

"Guys. It was a stressful time for me, yes. But that tear? It was a happy one. Think of it as a diamond forged from years of blood, sweat, falls, tears, and ice packs."

"You're trying to make me feel better," Mom says. "You don't have to, honey. I know I was wrong."

"I remember . . . I was thinking about how much I loved flying across the ice at that exact moment." I slowly let go of Gracie as she lets go of the chair, stretches her arms out, and balances. "And then I caught a judge smiling at me, and happiness bloomed inside me. Not just because my spiral made her smile, but because I was enjoying myself. I remembered I actually like skating."

"Like or liked?" Mom asks.

"Like," I say, smiling.

Out of her spiral, Gracie eyes the video and says, "Look, Madz. You're spinning so fast you look blurry." She scurries to a wide-open part of the floor, imitates the spin, and stumbles.

"Careful, Gracie," Mom says.

The music stops with my final pose, and the screen fades around the edges until all that's left is a still of me, posing in an oval bubble. An invisible hand writes underneath it "Madz Monroe, Final Freestyle Test" and the date. Gallagher claps, and Dad, Mom, and Gracie join in.

"All those years you invested in skating," Mom says. "You did it. You passed all of the tests." She hugs me. "I'm happy Will was there for you." Who would have thought our scruffy, young landscaper was such a gem?

<hr>

IN MADZ'S Hall of Fame, Gracie struggles to pick out a dress for her test and tryouts. She's torn between the red dress I wore for my salsa routine and the purple one I used for a maneuvers test.

"Wear both," I say. "One at a time, of course. The salsa one goes well with your freestyle-test music, and the purple one is perfect for tryouts. It's comfortable and looks great on you. You'll stand out." I open a drawer and pull out an unused pair of blade covers. I thought they were too pretty to use and get dirty.

"They're so puffy," Gracie says.

"Why don't you put them on your new skates? It's very important to protect your blades. If they're dull or burred, you won't be able to hold a good edge."

Gracie nods. We hang her dresses on a wall hook. "This is your section of the wall. Never wait until the last minute to get your skating stuff together for a test, a competition, or a tryout. The stress could affect your performance. Tights. Do you have a pair of tights with no runs or holes?"

"No. I have two pairs, and both have runs *and* holes."

I open another drawer, where I have unopened packages of them in a size I'm sure will fit her. I hang a package on the hook with her dresses. Then, I find matching hair scrunchies and hang them on the hook. "See how it's done?"

"Yeah. Thank you."

"Why do you look sad?"

"My tryout for ice theater is at SuperEdge, right?"

"Yup."

"What if the people there hate me like they do at the other rink?"

"They don't hate you. They just don't get you. Don't forget, you did scare them every time you busted out a scream."

A devilish smile grows on her face.

I point at her. "*That* is not nice. And SuperEdge won't put up with it. Be like Nathan. He's scarier when he's quiet."

"Okay, but those kids I scared deserved it. Whenever Will wasn't there, they would tell me I was weird and to get out of their way when I wasn't in their way. One told the proctor I should skate on a retarded session, which doesn't even exist." She sits and hugs her legs.

What is wrong with people? I sit next to her. "Gracie. There will always be haters out there. When they come your way, remember this: whether you're at SuperEdge or anywhere else, you have allies. Nathan, one of the best coaches in the country, has your back. Joao, one of the best skaters in the country, has your back. Will, my parents, and I have your back."

She rests her head on her knees. "Okay."

"Oh, and guess what?" I stand and rush to a wall of pictures. "If you make ice theater and keep trying hard and progressing, you could get a job as a teacher's assistant during group lessons." I point to a picture of me assistant-teaching a group lesson. "SuperEdge always needs help with the little kids in the learn-to-skate program."

Her eyes open wide, and she stands. "The coaches would let me help teach?"

"Of course. But you have to be a role model. You can't randomly yell or grunt, or whatever that thing was that you and Joao did."

She does it.

"How the heck do you do it, anyway?" I imitate her and grab my burning throat. "Ow."

Gracie smiles. "When your throat's better, I'll teach you. Joao does it the best."

"Gracie. Dear. De-grunt yourself. You're human, not a gorilla."

Gracie drops to the floor, laughing, holding her belly, and that's when I realize Joao hit the proverbial nail on the head:

humor is the key to reaching her. One more thing to love about her. And like about Joao.

"Let's go upstairs," I say. "You have an early morning appointment with your skate guy, remember?"

"You mean your skate guy."

"Yes, but now he's yours too."

Gracie looks in the mirror. "I have a skate guy."

THIRTY

Before putting on her skates at SuperEdge Sunday, Gracie tells Will to take his mother out of her backpack. Eventually, Mrs. Cruz will be buried in a forest, but not today. Gracie wants her mother present for her test and ice-theater tryouts. The container of ashes sits on Will's lap.

"So awkward," he says.

"Just keep telling yourself it's part of Gracie's healing process," I say. In a way, I think it's part of Will's, too, because he stares at me for a few seconds and then cracks a joke.

"I'm a human hearse," he says, covering his eyes, shaking his head, laughing.

Lindsey climbs the bleachers and squeezes between Will and me, forcing Nathan, Aunt Elaine, and me to slide to our left and shrinking the space between each person. I anticipated social-distancing issues. For that reason, I'm wearing an N-95 mask and planning my escape to an open area. What's annoying is Lindsey had no problem staying away from me for months, yet she's all over Will.

"Hold this a sec," he says, placing his mother on my lap. He pulls out Gracie's test form to show Lindsey, pointing to where it says Gracie passed the elementary freestyle test.

Will recorded the test while I watched Gracie through a lobby window. After she finished, Will beamed like a proud father. "I'm so proud of her," he said to me. We gave her a bouquet of flowers, and Mom and Dad gave her a membership to SuperEdge.

"I appreciate what you did to help make this happen," Will says to Lindsey, their eyes on Gracie's test results.

Nathan and I share a glance, and Nathan rolls his eyes.

"My pleasure," Lindsey says. "Isn't it nice how Gracie brought us all together?" She waves to me and leans into Will, her voice an angelic tone I've never heard come out of her mouth before.

"I can't," Nathan mumbles to me. He stands and waves his finger at Lindsey. "None of us would be here if Madz didn't ask me for help. I'm not tooting my own horn, but asking me for help had to be quite difficult for her ego." He nods to me, prodding me for validation.

"Yes, very difficult." I mirror his constant nodding and reluctantly continue speaking, sensing what he wants me to admit. "Especially after walking out on my lesson with you and . . ."

He raises his brows and tilts his head, egging me to finish the statement. I wince, instead, from the painful embarrassment he's about to inflict upon me.

"Go on. Say it, Madz. Writing a manifesto on the locker-room mirror in lipstick." His voice rises. "What did it say?" And rises. "Why are we doing this to ourselves? What are we here for?"

Cringing, I mumble, "Something like that."

Will leans back, our eyes meet behind Lindsey's head, and he says, "You wrote a manifesto in lipstick?"

"Indeed she did, Will. Indeed she did," Nathan says. He waves his pointer at me. "Touché."

If he's defending me, he has a weird way of doing it.

"I'd be lying," he says, "if I said you didn't inspire me to think about what I was doing here at this rink, Madz, what the whole point was to my being here."

"You went into the girls' locker room?" I ask.

"Don't get your feathers in a ruffle. I did it while the girls were on the ice, skating on the session following the one you walked out on. They'd swarmed around each other on the rink, buzzing about what you wrote, so I went in."

"He made all of his students write a response to it," Lindsey says, rolling her eyes, "and refused to give them a lesson until they passed it in. I had to do the freaking assignment before I could become his student." She nudges me. "Thanks a lot."

I look up at Nathan. "They must hate me."

"Some probably do, but the question you posed commanded serious reflection. What's the point of being here if you don't know why you're here? Why should I waste my time coaching kids who don't know why they're here?"

"I wrote that thinking skating was killing me. I didn't know I had—"

"Doesn't matter. Others have thought it; they just didn't have the nuggets to put it down in bright-red lipstick. I overheard another one of my students ponder the same question at a test session. She was talking to another skater as they waited their turn. She was unaware I was within hearing range."

"Spy," I say.

"Maybe. But here's the point: You spotlighted a question skaters sometimes ask themselves, especially when they're spending their lives at the rink, training, falling, and hurting. If they don't know why they're doing it, they might never learn the sport's deeper lessons that build character and prepare them for life. Or at least, they may never connect future successes to their training here.

"Madz humbled herself and asked me for help for no other reason than to keep a promise." He looks at Lindsey. "This wasn't *mandatory* volunteer work for her."

Will recoils, furrows his brow, and looks at Lindsey.

"If skating with me enabled that ethic in Madz, then I'm totally good with having worked with"—he turns, points his finger at me—"you. In fact, it's why I didn't think twice about helping you."

He smiles. "With that said . . ." He sits, leans forward, and turns to Lindsey. "Yes, Lindsey. Of course we wouldn't be here together if it weren't for Gracie. She's executing a plan. She's holding up her end of the bargain. Commitment. Isn't that why we're all here today?" He looks at me with a single raised eyebrow and jerks his head toward Lindsey.

She's showing Will pictures of herself on her social media account.

"Here she is," Will says, just as I think we wouldn't be here without him, thanks to a legendary deal he made on behalf of his sister. Because he was determined to make Gracie's skating wishes come true. "Can we switch sides, Lindsey?" He stands, squeezes between her and me, and sits. Gracie positions herself in the center of the ice with her group.

I pass Will his mother. The music plays, and Gracie pushes off, three-turns to a back crossover—crap. She fell.

"What happened?" Nathan asks, standing.

"Is she hurt? She never sits that long after a fall," Will says, standing.

"Her blade," I say. Drowning in a sea of skaters continuing the routine, Gracie looks at me, her eyes lighting up like full moons at midnight. Pleasedon'tscreampleasedon'tscreampleasedon't—"Nathan. Go help her. Tell them to stop. They'll trip over her."

He doesn't have to. The music stops, and the coach directing tryouts—the gingerbread-tea-toting Mrs. Claus look-alike—checks Gracie's blade. The coach pulls Gracie up and off the ice as Gracie balances on one foot. I was afraid her skates would conk out, but Mom taught me to always be prepared. I grab my tote bag and climb down the bleachers. Nathan and Will follow me down.

"I've got this," I say to them. "I know what's wrong." The blade on the skate she can't stand on is askew. The sole is moldy and soft. I'm not surprised the blade screws lost their grip; her test pushed them to the limit. I couldn't talk her into wearing the new ones. Although our skate guy made sure they fit her like a glove, Gracie insisted on testing in her old ones. She kept saying, "I know how they work."

I pull off my mask, sit next to Gracie, and unzip my bag. "Are you hurt?"

"No." She huffs. "You were right. I should have used my new—"

I pull out her new skates. "Hurry. Unlace those things." I

ask Mrs. Claus, "She can go back out, right?" *Please*, I mouth to her.

"Make it snappy." She sips her tea and skates over to the girls on the ice, who return to their starting positions.

I take over unlacing Gracie's skates, throw on the new ones, and lace them. I pull Gracie up and say, "Jump up and down in them a couple of times." She does, and I practically push her onto the ice. "Go get 'em."

She skates cautiously, gradually picks up speed, and stops in her proper place. She's worn them around my house, in my skating room, so she's gotten to "know" them a little.

The music starts. I stay put, holding my breath, extra challenging because my lungs crave air after being smothered by the heavy mask. I toss it in the trash.

"You're officially a skating mom," Will says, standing behind me, holding the container of ashes.

"Shh." I give Gracie a thumbs-up. Shivering, I cross my arms to hold in body heat while the new refrigeration system breathes down my neck.

Will wraps his arm around me and rubs my arm, warming me.

I fix my eyes on Gracie. "No wonder my mother's nerves were strung so tight when I competed or tested."

"It's amazing she can concentrate after everything she's been through. I think it's a gift autism gave her. That and her honesty." As he watches Gracie, his face tenses, mirroring my sentiments.

Nathan put in a good word for her, but she won't be put on the team if she unravels. "It's not the end of the world if she doesn't make it," I say to him. "She can always try out for ice theater next year."

"I don't want to be the one to tell her that."

Entering her spiral, Grace lifts her leg higher than the other candidates. She glides across the ice, smiling. The upbeat music calls for the expression, but I doubt she's acting. Nathan gives me a thumbs-up. Next, she goes into a spin, centers it, and I'm so proud of her. I grip the arm cocooning me and say to Will, "She has the best spin. See how centered it is?"

"She's better than half of them."

I hate to break from his embrace, but I do and say, "Let's pack up her old skates and get back to the bleachers. I don't want her new friends to think she has helicopter siblings."

Back on the bleachers, we sit in front of Nathan. "She'll probably be in this group for a year or two," he says. "If she keeps up the good work, she'll move up a level."

Joao approaches us. "She's doing great in those new skates."

"She's a good skater," Aunt Elaine says, leaning forward, watching intently. "What a pretty dress. She looks beautiful in purple with those pink cheeks of hers. Lovely. Just lovely."

"Looks like you've proven yourself as a coach," Will says, high-fiving Joao. "You've got the job."

"I'll give you the family discount," Joao says.

"Thanks. My budget could use the help."

The group finishes their routine with a series of single jumps and a final scratch spin. Mrs. Claus gives Nathan the thumbs up.

"She did it," I say, smiling.

Gracie heads to the locker room, signaling me to join her. I hold up my pointer finger, not wanting to enter a packed locker room.

After most of the candidates leave, Will walks me around

the rink. We sit at a table by the snack bar. Aunt Elaine comes out of the main office and sits with us.

She hands Will a receipt. "This is my present to Gracie for passing her test and earning a spot on the ice-theater team. I paid her cast-member dues. It covers traveling and costume costs."

"Thank you." His brow furrows. "I had money put aside for it."

She rests her hands on his. "Spend it on yourself for a change."

"Excuse me." He walks out of the rink. I follow him outside and sit next to him on a bench. "It's always been Gracie and me. Now everyone's . . . involved. As if I can't handle the situation. My mother's a bunch of ashes now, but in a way she's been dead for a long time. The urn just makes it official. My sister and I are in no different a situation than we were before."

I think hard before I speak, wanting to be honest without being offensive. "Your situation *is* different. You have friends who care about you and your sister, and you have extended family. Your aunt seems to really care. It's okay to accept help; no one will judge you. We all know everything you've done for your sister."

"I don't think anyone will ever know everything. It goes far beyond the financial aspect of taking care of her. There's a bond there, and if you think it's been easier for me not having her around, you're wrong. I haven't said it to anyone else because I know Gracie is safe. And she's distracted from the fact her mother bailed on her."

I rest my hand on his, hoping my touch, gentle and warm, relays I get what he says, I feel for him, and I plan to stick with him. "Gracie isn't completely distracted. She knows her mother bailed, and she had a good cry over it." My mind flashes back to the image of her face, tragedy written all over it, as we hid behind the parlor palm.

"Sad tears or angry ones?"

"Sad. Really sad. Being with me and my parents didn't make her forget her mother. Just as no distance between you and Gracie, and no financial arrangements that lighten the burden on you, will take away how important you are to her."

Five minutes later, we're back inside. Lindsey peeks her head out of the locker room and signals me to come in.

I walk into the familiar space. It's empty except for Lindsey and Gracie. Lindsey waves her hand toward the mirror, and I face it. A message, written in red lipstick, has replaced my mini-manifesto: "We [heart] Madz." On the counter beneath the mirror sits a card. I open it and find hand-written names and get-well wishes. They aren't from the skaters who just tried out with Gracie. I don't know them. The names and notes are from the skaters I spent years training with. Skaters I grew up with here. My friends.

"Are you mad?" Gracie says.

"Why?"

"Because they found out. You look like you're in shock."

I was desperate to hide my illness. Maybe I needed to; maybe I didn't. In the end, though, doing so created a void deep in my soul. But these kind words, hearts, and XOs fill that empty space and lift my spirit to a better place.

"No, I'm not mad, Gracie. I'm happy I have friends who care."

By keeping my friends in the dark, I gave myself space to rest, space to look and feel miserable without having to explain why. Chelsea was the only person who could truly understand, the one person I could be totally comfortable with.

Maybe I did my friends a favor by not telling them. It allowed them to focus on their jumps instead of confronting an ugly truth that Chelsea and I knew all too well: young people get cancer, and nothing short of a miracle can change that. Then again, perhaps my friends are wiser than I think. A few might have already known a kid who had cancer, and one of these XOs could have been written by a fellow cancer survivor.

A smile blossoms as I read the precious collection of signatures and comments.

"I couldn't hold it in anymore," Lindsey says. "I told one person, and the next thing I knew, everyone was asking me questions, talking about it in here, saying they wanted to do something for you. I thought you'd never speak to me again if you found out I broke my promise to keep quiet. But you're almost cured now, right? So we're good? I'm thinking we are because Nathan hasn't dumped me yet."

"This is really . . . special." I hug her.

"I've been a terrible friend these past few months," she says. "I wasn't sure what to say or if you'd get mad at me if I said the wrong thing. I looked back at my texts to you and cringed over how I'd blabbed about how great things were while you were struggling through harsh treatments." She blots her tears with her sleeve. "Honestly, I was kind of glad you didn't want to acknowledge being sick. I thought that gave me a pass to ignore it. And when you stopped texting me, I followed your lead."

"Well, then, I have to forgive you. My lead wasn't exactly exemplary." Growing up, we learn how to write, how to work through math problems, and how to figure out the main point of a paragraph. *How to deal with teen cancer* isn't on the syllabus.

She pulls out of the hug and touches my "hair." "This isn't yours, is it? I mean—"

"No. It's someone else's hair. *Was* someone else's hair. It's mine now, at least until my follicles snap out of their coma."

"It's pretty. I love the beanie too." She sits on a bench. "Sit with me." I do, and she says, "Can I be honest about something else?"

"Shoot."

"I've always felt proud to have you as a friend, and I'm grateful you stayed my friend when, on occasion, I wasn't my best self. When you walked out on your lesson with Na—"

"I'm not proud of how I left. It was rude."

"No. Listen. When you left, you thought you were doing the right thing for yourself, for your body. That took guts. Everyone's so regimented around here—skaters, our parents, our coaches. Disrupting the regimen to do something for your-self? That's groundbreakingly brave. Inspirational."

"I was frustrated and scared. I had the wrong idea as to why I was feeling crappy. It didn't necessarily take guts."

"Yes, it did. I still skated at SuperEdge, though. When you stopped texting me, I looked back at my texts to you and concluded you didn't want to be friends with me for one of two possible reasons: I either reminded you of what you wanted to move on from or I was a painful reminder of the world you had to leave because you were sick."

"Sounds like even you were tempted to believe Nathan's white lie about why I wasn't at the rink with Gracie."

"Ah, that's right. You were too upset about him not taking you back as a student. I think I did convince myself it was true." We giggle.

"I can hear you guys," Gracie says. "You shouldn't laugh

about Nathan lying to me. That's rude. In case you didn't know, I only forgave him for it because he helped me and because Madz forced him to lie." Gracie zips up her skate bag and stands. "I'm going out to see Will."

"Gracie, wait," I say, scurrying to her. I hug her. "Congratulations."

"Nice job," Lindsey says, high-fiving her.

"Thanks, Lindsey, but just so you know, I'm Madz's best friend, not you."

Lindsey looks at me, and I shrug.

"Gracie," I say, "will you tell Will I'll be right there?"

"Yup." She leaves.

"Is it wrong that I'm totally jealous about you and Will?" Lindsey asks.

"No, you're right to be jealous. He's gorgeous, and he's an awesome person." I look at the card again, at all the signatures.

"Every one of them wanted to text you. They wanted to video-chat with you. They also respected your wishes."

"They didn't even look at me at the picnic."

"One, they didn't know you'd just found out you were sick; two, that was a legit case of guilt-by-association fear. Your scandalous exit was still fresh, and so was the assignment Nathan gave them. But when they did find out you'd been sick and that you'd be here tonight, they said, 'F-it. She's getting a card whether she likes it or not.'"

"I'm glad you guys said 'F-it.'"

THIRTY-ONE
NINE MONTHS LATER

S ometimes I wonder if I did more harm than good by not telling my friends I had cancer. I hurt Will and Gracie, and by shutting out peers I'd skated with for years, I think I hurt them. Did I short-change myself? Could I have gotten through my treatments any easier by adding more people to my special little circle of trust? Would it have changed my story? Chelsea's?

I couldn't fool her. She could read on my face what she herself had felt at one point or another. I wouldn't have had the strength to fake feeling good around my friends during the worst days of my treatments. And then there were the germs to consider.

I'm pretty sure there's no right or wrong way to get through cancer, just as there's no particular way to accept death or any life-changing event life throws at us. But now's the time. Now's the time I share how Chelsea got through pain and sorrow, how she managed to pluck joy from the field of weeds that overran her life. Now's the time I share with everyone watching what they missed by not knowing her and what I gained from knowing her.

When Nathan asked me months ago to skate in tonight's SuperEdge show, he said, "I have an assignment for you. By the end of it, you'll know why you worked so hard in skating." He said the club planned to donate the show's proceeds to a good cause: Haven Shore's Wishing Well, a program for pediatric cancer patients.

I didn't want to let him down, but I was afraid he'd set an unrealistic goal for me. I was afraid to commit because Life and I had some trust-building to do. I was afraid I wouldn't be strong enough to perform, afraid I would let down the patients of Haven Shore's pediatric clinic. My clinic. Chelsea's clinic.

You see, kids like us aren't a cause. We're reluctant warriors fighting daily battles in our own unique wars. My performance would need to be personal. When I decided to skate in memory of Chelsea, she became the wind beneath my wings—the wind that fed the desire to represent her, to skate for her, to remind the audience this angel existed.

Nathan hands me a tissue. I blow my nose, and he takes the crinkled mess from me. I love him for that. He did it when I competed too.

"I don't want to let her down," I say. "I don't want to let her parents down. The song doesn't tell everything about her. It doesn't do her enough justice." Nathan's partner, Craig, is in the music business. He and I wrote the lyrics, and Craig's friend put them to music. It's personal and special, but can any song truly sum up a life and all its struggles?

"Do her justice through your skating," Nathan says. "Show what the song doesn't tell. Harness the love, Madz. Your love for Chelsea and all kids suffering through what she went through. What you went through. You're strong enough to do that now."

The announcer's voice echoes through the arena. "Ladies and gentlemen, tonight, as we raise money for Haven Shore Cancer Institute's Wishing Well program, we celebrate children who have fought, are fighting, or will fight this tragic disease. Please welcome Madelyn Monroe, a gold-tested member of SuperEdge, a Northeast sectional bronze medalist, and a cancer survivor. She's skating in honor of six-year-old Chelsea Hart, who recently lost her battle with cancer."

Deep breath in. I blow it out and push against the ice, stroke, stroke, stroking to the center, concentration dulling the roar of applause. I pose, crossing my hands over my chest, looking down, focusing on a minute section of the ice. In the silence, my spirit joins Chelsea's. When the music starts, the butterfly I held before her eyes takes wing with me.

> *So little, so sweet—*
> *Butterfly among bees—*
> *You're tangled in weeds that grow inside*
> *And tether your wings so you can't fly.*

Tell them who she was, I think, unclutching my chest, stretching my arms out, stroking, three-turning, setting up for my first jump—a double flip—then hopping into a flying camel spin.

> *You're fighting for a life you've yet to live,*
> *Dying for a breath you long to breathe:*
> *The air outside these walls, unleashed—*

Outside these walls, where you might fall,
But at least
You'll see stars shimmering,
Heaven, and angel wings glimmering
Like the butterfly, the one that caught your eye
In the garden.

As I glide through my routine, my arms flow with the music as if I'm conducting it myself, conducting the story of Chelsea. She's with me—I feel it—as I pick up speed and enter a spiral. I lean forward, extend my leg, and lift it high while stretching out my arms. My hands flutter like butterfly wings as the wind weaves through my new curls and I breeze across the ice, thinking, *This is what I trained for, this feeling, this warm, joyful sense. I'm an artist animating the still.* I've brought Chelsea back for a moment, and she's flying, the wind beneath her wings powered by an abundance of love.

Then, I no longer flutter but launch, confident in my newfound strength, channeling the child who understands and accepts her fate but still tries to live. Even in pain she's determined to experience joy—Russian split—if only for a moment. That one last moment before she dies.

Some of us fight and win,
But in the struggle, we hurt and spin—
Taking toxic hits, crying in the pits,
Wondering, Will this ever end?

But you, who fought the battle and lost the war,
Whose soul Hell rattled but never tore—
Who never made seven,

Who flies in Heaven—

You shared a smile with me,
And in my misery,
I found a friend.

Arms spread, shoulders back, chin up, my edges grip the ice as I fly across it, but I may as well be twirling across the sky. I am Chelsea and I am me, pain-free. I am all the kids who grew wings and said, "Today the sky is mine, the wind and the air are mine, and time doesn't matter because I'm finally free." We're angels, we're people, foot-working, spiraling, twizzling, split-jumping, three-turning into a triple—yes, triple—toe loop, flying higher than we ever imagined we could.

Break out; break free
Beyond the Sea of Dreams—
Dreamt but will never be—
The Sea of Mothers and Fathers
Whose hurt you feel,
The Sea of Sisters and Brothers
Who fight the will
To flee to a place pain-free.

Break out; break free
To the stars, shimmering;
To Heaven, your angel wings glimmering
Like the butterfly,
The one that caught your eye
In the garden.

Some of us fight and win,
But in the struggle, we swirl and spin—
Taking toxic hits, crying in the pits,
Wondering, Will this ever end?

But you, who fought the battle and lost the war,
Whose soul Hell rattled but never tore—
Who never made seven,
Who flies in Heaven—

You shared a smile with me,
And in my misery,
I found a friend.

The music slows, Chelsea's strength weakens, and the angel, this child angel, bows to her maker, blows a kiss to the world, and looks up to her destination. Untangled from the weeds, our beloved child stretches her wings and flies beyond the walls that confined her, alive again.

So little, so sweet—
Butterfly among bees—
God carries you outside these walls,
Where you don't fall.

Your wings untether.
You're light as a feather,
Flying to the stars, glimmering;
To Heaven, your angel wings shimmering

Like the butterfly,

The one who flutters by in a memory
And shares a smile with me—
My friend.

The music ends, but the love, the purest kind she radiates, is indelible. Filled with gratitude, I rise from my own bed of weeds, free and winged like a butterfly launching from its dark cocoon. My destination is up in the air, but my options are limitless because of where I stand now: this heavenly place I struggled to get to. Here, what people think doesn't matter as much as how they make a difference for the better in their own unique ways. Here, I rediscover my love of skating because this is where the answer lives, the answer to the question I posed in lipstick months ago.

"Thank you, Chelsea," I say to the rafters while the audience stands and claps. I bow, then blow a kiss to her parents, who sit in a "special guests" penalty box with my parents, a Haven Shore PR representative, and Candy. I blow a kiss to my parents, who blow kisses to me. I blow a kiss to the roaring crowd throwing flowers and stuffed animals onto the ice.

A little girl skates onto the ice and hands me a bouquet of flowers. Dodging the mines of gifts on the ice, I skate to Theresa and hand her the bouquet. She hugs me hard. When she pulls away, I pick up as many flowers and teddy bears as my arms can hold, blow another kiss to the audience, and skate backstage. Several skaters rush out from there to clear off what I couldn't pick up.

As I place my armful of gifts next to the boards, Nathan throws my sweater onto my shoulders, but I don't feel cold. I'm swirling in a whirlwind of emotion I've never felt before, and it feels . . . warm. He hugs me, squashing the small bouquet of flowers and teddy bear I kept. "Your best skate ever. Your jumps were huge. You could've easily gotten a quad out of that triple toe. Just one more—"

"Thank you, Nathan. You're more special than any of those people out there will ever know, except maybe Craig."

He places his finger over his lips. "Shh. I have a reputation to keep."

I skate to the boards, past the finale lineup, from which Gracie's hand reaches out and high-fives mine. She's bossing around the little kids, telling them where to stand. That's her job. She's assisting their coach.

I stretch my guards onto my blades and leave the rink.

IN THE DRESSING ROOM, I sweep my fingers along Chelsea's signature, slip my skate back into my bag, and pull out the infamous red salsa lipstick. Leaning against the counter, pressing my lipstick against the mirror, I write "Fly in peace, Chelsea," then draw a heart with wings and leave the flowers and teddy bear on the counter underneath. As I head out, the door behind me closes with a determined echo that sounds throughout the dimly lit hall.

I've never missed the finale of a show I was in. I'd savor every second of the lights, the cheers, and the laughs with my peers. Now, I embrace the muffled sounds of the final performance: the bass thumping the wall, the distant applause. As much as I appreciate the warmth the audience radiated, I'd prefer not to drown in a sea of strangers and germs. Not yet, anyway.

Light beams at the end of the hall, where Will waits before

the "Performers Only" sign. Butterflies still flutter in my stomach when I see him.

He greets me with a smile, a hug, and I breathe him in because I can. Because my counts are normal, I'm strong and unmasked, and I don't care about germs when I'm pressed against him.

"Your parents and Gallagher said they'll wait for Gracie and meet us at the restaurant. My father can't go; he's working the night shift—oh." He pulls away and hands me a rose. "Not much compared to what the audience threw you."

I close my eyes and sniff the rose.

"What did you do with all of those stuffed animals?" he asks.

"Donated them. The Haven Shore rep said she'd take care of it. I asked her to give the flowers to the staff."

He wraps his arms around me again. "I liked watching you skate. Do you think you can give me a few lessons? I'm sure we can work out a deal."

"Deals can get pretty complicated," I say, my face moving in on his as he pulls me closer. "I—"

"..."

A kiss is like a spiral, a beautiful, comfortable break. Except your arms spread out only to wrap around the person you love, who anchors you while your mind swirls and whose fingers are the wind running through your hair. As Will runs his through mine, I'm sure he knows I've already accepted the deal.

NOTES

Chapter 26

1. part of Psalms 23:4 (King James Version of the Bible)

AUTHOR'S NOTE

Thank you for reading *The Beauty of a Spiral*. Writing this story was deeply personal because I, like Madz, battled cancer as a teenager. I was diagnosed with stage IIA Hodgkin's lymphoma at age eighteen, and at one point during my radiation treatments, no medication could quell my nausea. (The high-dose radiation I received in 1982 is no longer standard treatment because of its concerning long-term effects.)

While waiting for my treatments, I sometimes sat with children much younger than I was. I didn't know what type of cancer they had, but I could tell from their scars, radiation markings, and lumps that it wasn't the same as mine. Sitting among them, I felt lucky to have gotten a cancer I imagined was "easier" than theirs, given my doctor had described mine as a curable "inconvenience."

As mentioned on the copyright page, this book is a fictitious work, the story a product of my imagination. Scenes that mention real places or things are fictional. All characters, the places they go to, and the events in their lives are not real. Any similarity to an actual person, business establishment, club, facility, or event is coincidental.

Important to note, I don't intend to provide advice or influence health-care decisions via this story. If you have questions about cancer or another condition mentioned in this book, discuss them with a parent, guardian, or a trusted medical expert or therapist, depending on your age and circumstances.

Current and future treatments for Hodgkin's lymphoma may or may not include drugs in the ABVD protocol Madz receives. Although those drugs are real, and some real people may have received any or all of them, Madz's treatment scenario is hypothetical and, again, employed fictitiously. Consider, too, that new discoveries can lead to changes in treatment protocols.

Because Madz's hyperosmia makes her super sensitive to smells, she gets extra nauseous from her infusions. Madz doesn't represent all people or anyone in particular receiving any or all of the drugs in the ABVD protocol or diagnosed with hyperosmia, Hodgkin's lymphoma, or both, just as her skater friends and her coach do not represent any particular individual in the figure-skating world.

For the record, my two daughters figure-skated for years, and from pre-teen to fifty, I skated as well. We met terrific people, and despite the occasional "hard fall," we enjoyed the sport.

Fiction can reflect reality. And in reality, life sometimes deals young people cancer diagnoses, thrusting them into wars where their bodies are the battlefield. Individual experiences may vary but are bound by common threads, like those woven throughout *The Beauty of a Spiral* and my own personal, very real story. Such themes highlight the courage and perseverance of young cancer patients while spotlighting the compassion of caregivers, the love of family, and the kindness of friends, all of which make the sweetest lemonade from the lemons served.

ACKNOWLEDGMENTS

Thanks to . . .

My family: Janelle, whose spiral is so beautiful that it would even inspire Madz. Brooke, a talented novel writer who let me bounce things off her as I created and polished the story. Jimmy, for his love, support, and loyalty.

My mother, for reading the story, encouraging me to publish it, and for being an awesome mom in general. Also, my late father, for taking me to the hospital countless times before I was finally diagnosed with Hodgkin's disease and for breaking the news to me with reassuring strength when I woke up from anesthesia after having my neck lump biopsied.

Laurie Chittenden, developmental editor, whose thoughtful insights helped me strengthen the story and whose encouraging words motivated me.

"Miss Patty," long-time figure skater and coach (who can still knock out a beautiful spiral), my friend, and my go-to for information about current figure-skating trends and happenings. Her perseverance inspires.

Katie Jolley, for working diligently and patiently on my book cover and for her work on the Ponderlit logo.

Kimberly Dias, NP, for her dedication to oncology nursing and for answering a host of questions that helped me fact-check myself.

Beta readers Alexia, Amber Lilyquist, and Katelyn Rothney, for their story dives and engaging comments. Also, thanks to everyone else who critiqued a few chapters or the entire book.

Ana Joldes, for her meticulous proofreading.

Health-care providers who have treated me over the years (Boston's best), for keeping me alive this long, and the ancillary team members who greeted me with a smile. Furthermore, all health-care providers and empathetic personnel, for your essential work.